BEATING

DIABETES

HOW TO DEFEAT THE HORRORS OF TYPE 2 DIABETES

PAUL D KENNEDY

Dedication

To diabetics or pre-diabetics everywhere in the hopes that they may find some use of this book.

Publisher's note

While every possible effort has been made to ensure that the information contained in this book is accurate, the author, editor and publisher cannot accept responsibility for any errors or omissions, however caused.

No responsibility for any loss or damage occasioned by any person acting or refraining from acting as a result of the material in this publication can be accepted by the author, editor or publisher.

Apart from any fair dealing for the purposes of research or private study, or criticism or review, this publication may only be reproduced, stored or transmitted, in any form or by any means, with the prior permission in writing of the author.

Enquiries concerning reproduction outside these terms should be sent to the author at:

paul@beating-diabetes.com

Copyright 2013 Paul D Kennedy

Paul D Kennedy is an international business consultant, researcher, writer and publisher. He is a graduate of Trinity College, Dublin, and a Fellow of the Chartered Association of Certified Accountants.

Beating Diabetes is based on Paul Kennedy's personal experience in avoiding the horrendous consequences of type 2 diabetes. You can contact him at:

Email: paul@beating-diabetes.com

Websites
www.beating-diabetes.com
ww.thornislandpublishing.com
www.consulting-services.eu
www.writingservices.eu
www.kuwaitbusinessguide.com
www.kuwait1990.com
www.arabic-tales.com

Checklists & Reference Materials

The last section of *Beating Diabetes* contains several checklists and some other reference material. Readers who are determined to beat their diabetes would find these very useful. The material is available online for downloading as a PDF file.

Just go to www.beating-diabetes.com and look for DOWNLOADS in the right side-bar. Click on 'Signup and download Checklists & References' which will take you to a sign-up form. After signing up you will receive an email with a link to the PDF booklet *Checklists & References* which you can open and then save to your hard disk.

Weekly Blog

Paul Kennedy writes and publishes a blog on topics of interest for type 2 diabetics. To put yourself on the mailing list for these articles, just to go to www.beating-diabetes.com and click on SIGN-UP.

Privacy policy: please note that we will never share your email address with anyone at all. You can read our full privacy policy on our website: www.beating-diabetes.com.

Disclaimer and warning
From the author

I am not a medical doctor, not a nurse, not a medical scientist and not a dietician. Though I am an experienced business researcher, the only medical knowledge I have is the knowledge I have gained through reading books and browsing the internet.

Please note that all the information in *Beating Diabetes* is based on my personal experience or on what I obtained through research on the internet. As such, it may not be accurate or perhaps some of the concepts have been over-simplified. Nevertheless, this knowledge did help me devise a diet which I am using to beat my diabetes.

This book is not prescriptive and does not give advice. It describes the changes in life-style and diet I followed to beat my type 2 diabetes. The changes worked for me with tremendous results. Thus, they are likely to work for you too if you follow my example. However this is not guaranteed.

Before following the diet I am using, you should consult a qualified healthcare advisor, such as your doctor or diabetes clinic.

My Story

I am a diabetic. I have type 2 diabetes and there is no cure.

This condition has horrendous consequences. Diabetes will eventually damage my heart, kidneys, eyes and extremities. I could end up with gangrene in my legs which would then have to be amputated. The outlook is an early death ... slow, messy and painful ... unless I do something about it.

I did that something. And now I believe I have found a way to postpone the terrible future that type 2 diabetes holds for most people who suffer from it.

There is no cure, that's for sure. But there is a way you can beat diabetes and hold off its horrible outcomes, a way that's very easy and practical.

I was first diagnosed with borderline or early onset diabetes in 2001.

My condition gradually became worse until a few years ago when I researched what I could do to beat it.

My research proved very fruitful. All I had to do, I discovered, was to eliminate certain foods from what I was eating. I did so and my numbers (blood glucose, cholesterol and blood pressure levels) improved dramatically.

I also added a bit of daily exercise, though this does not seem to be crucial for beating diabetes. However exercise is important in controlling blood pressure.

I now feel a lot lighter, healthier and more energetic. And beating diabetes ... putting off the effects it was having on my body ... has improved my prospects of living to a ripe old age.

My solution involves no costly medicines, no weird diets, and no strenuous exercises ... no big deal at all.

You too can probably beat your type-2 diabetes with nothing more than a simple change in diet, a cheap yet effective solution.

You don't even have to exercise much at all.

And food tastes so much better.

Here's my story ...

I enjoyed pretty good health until 1990, despite the high pressure lifestyle of an international management consultant and a mainly fast-food diet along with forty (two packs) of cigarettes (sometimes more) a day.

I was living in Kuwait where I was working as a senior consultant with a well-known regional bank when Iraq invaded that country in August 1990.

Like every other Westerner in Kuwait, when Saddam announced that we were to be rounded up as hostages and used as human shields to protect Iraq's key military and industrial installations, I immediately went into hiding. As you can imagine, the situation was extremely stressful.

I discovered later that, as an Irish citizen, I was able to move around Kuwait and Iraq. I organised the distribution of food for Westerners in hiding, undertook minor intelligence-gathering activities and a few trivial acts of resistance. But all that is another story (see www.kuwait1990.com).

I finally got to Jordan just before Christmas in 1990. I came down with some sort of flu and went to a doctor. My blood pressure was very high. I had developed hypertension. The fear, tension and stress I experienced in Kuwait and Iraq had a significant adverse effect on my long-term health.

Back in Kuwait after liberation, my hypertension began to slowly worsen and I began taking Tenoret, a combination of atenolol and chlorthalidone, to control my blood pressure. At the time I was a jack-of-all-trades, doing management consulting during the daytime and moon-lighting on the local radio station as a presenter and writer. I eventually became a publisher of guide-books and magazines, an extremely sedentary occupation.

I had just launched a consumer magazine when I noticed swollen ridges on the back of my tongue. As I was smoking two packs of cigarettes a day at that time, I got a bad scare and thought I had throat cancer. But no, it was diabetes, type 2 early onset diabetes.

The medical advice I got in Kuwait (all free at the government's expense) was excellent. As a border-line case, I was told that I needed to control my diet to eliminate sugar and fat as far as possible to prevent the disease from developing. If I'd had the wit to follow that advice I would probably still be at the early-onset stage of diabetes today.

Drinking tea without sugar was easy. Taking coffee without sugar was a real struggle. I used to love (still do) sweet sticky Turkish coffee. Without the sugar it was a different drink. But eventually I realised that the caffeine kick was just as good without the sugar and I was able to habituate myself successfully to sugar-free beverages. But, as regards diet control, that was about as far as I went.

I had been told to avoid cheese (unless it was fat-free) and to eat eggs (which are 50% fat) only once a week. Fat-free cheese tastes absolutely yucky and I never made the change-over, just reduced the amount of cheese I ate. Though I'd always been fond of eggs … sunny side up on toast, scrambled, omelettes … I managed to cut them down a bit, but not too much.

I still felt quite healthy. Life continued and the good advice I got faded from memory. The only thing that became a permanent feature of my diet at this stage was the elimination of sugar from my tea and coffee. I continued to smoke two packs a day. My blood glucose levels were checked twice a year and, not surprisingly, my blood sugar count gradually crept upwards.

Back in Ireland on a visit in March 2005 I experienced a sudden pain in my right leg, just above the knee, late at night. The pain persisted for about 20 minutes and then faded. When it was over I found that the muscles of my right leg were very stiff and I was hobbling when I tried to walk. I thought I had twisted a muscle around my knee.

At first I could only walk a few yards before my calf muscle seized up and I had to rest and wait a few minutes before hobbling on. Eventually my right calf eased up more and more and I was able to walk a hundred yards or so without having to pause. Believe it or not, it was about four months before I consulted a doctor! I had been lucky!

In fact, very lucky. I had a burst aneurism in my right leg … the artery that conveys blood down my leg had clotted in place just above the knee. If it had broken loose, it would have travelled up to my heart or brain and given me a massive heart attack or a stroke. I had escaped a life-threatening situation through no effort on my own part.

However the clot was preventing blood from flowing down below my knee so the muscles in my lower leg were being deprived of blood. This meant that I could only walk a few metres (yards) before the muscles seized up and I had to stop to allow them to recover.

The doctors explained that eventually the smaller veins in my leg would, provided I continued to walk as much as possible, enlarge and convey more blood to my lower leg. They did ... slowly ... and eight years later I can walk as far as I want before I have to pause for a rest, provided I stick to a slow pace.

The doctors also found another aneurism ... one that was about to pop ... just above my left knee. They did a by-pass, joining the artery to the blood vessels just below the knee. It went fine. But they also told me that I had peripheral vascular disease (PVD), meaning that my arteries were obstructed by plaque and that the blood supply to my feet (in particular) was very poor.

The plaque was due to fatty deposits building up over time in the blood vessels. PVD is essentially a life-style disease. It is caused by smoking, type 2 diabetes, high cholesterol levels, and hypertension. The causes of my PVD fitted that bill exactly.

I was advised repeatedly to give up smoking. So I cut down. I didn't give up. I was still being blasé and stupid about my health.

I was urged to get my diabetes and cholesterol levels under control. I began attending a local diabetes clinic. In addition to the Tenoret for my hypertension (blood pressure), I was prescribed Nu-Seals, a slow release aspirin, to reduce the risk of blood-clots forming, and Pravastatin, a statin which reduces the body's production of cholesterol, all to be taken daily.

But the diabetes clinic I began attending in 2005 went one better. They gave me some portable measurement equipment so that I was able to measure my blood glucose levels at home ... lancets for pricking my finger and test strips that I inserted into a little gauge before dipping the tip into the little bubble of blood on my pricked finger. The gauge gave a read-out of my glucose level. I began checking my blood sugar regularly and keeping records (the consultancy habit kicking in).

The clinic also gave me plenty of advice on my diet. I discovered later that this advice was based loosely on the diet recommended by the American Diabetes Association.

It involved cutting down on the overall quantities I eat and reducing my consumption of certain products. It was essentially a low carbohydrate diet, with reduced fruit consumption (due to the natural sugars in the fruit). I was not told to give up any foods at all, just to reduce the amounts I ate.

A pity! I found out later that the key to beating diabetes is to give up certain foods entirely and eat as much as you like of the rest. This is what worked for me anyway.

In the meantime, I followed the diet ... more or less. I avoided sweet foods, switched to low-fat milk and only had bacon, sausages, eggs, etc (the typical Irish 'fry') once a week.

But my weight still remained in the 'fat' range (my BMI was in the late 20s) but below 'obese' and my glucose levels continued to creep upwards.

The problems with my feet got gradually worse ... I was losing sensation in my left foot, and now and then my feet seemed to be on fire, at other times they felt frozen. I began experiencing tingles in my hands, signs of incipient neuropathy (problems with the nerve paths).

My health was slowly getting worse.

I finally gave up smoking 100% in 2008. It was a heck of a struggle. Only a confirmed smoker can appreciate the effort required to give up smoking. For years afterwards I chewed Nicorette ... a gum that delivers nicotine but avoids the ill-effects of the tar-and-carcinogens in cigarettes.

On a visit to the diabetes clinic in mid-2009 the doctors found that my blood glucose levels and other factors were no longer under proper control through my diet. I was put on Glucophage (metformin) to be taken twice a day to improve my body's sensitivity to the insulin my pancreas was producing.

Another medication, Coversyl (perindopril arginine), was added to my treatment. Coversyl is designed to help maintain blood pressure levels and I was prescribed it to improve the capacity of the veins in my feet.

So there I was in the summer of 2009, on five 'maintenance' drugs a day ... Tenoret, slow-release aspirin, Pravastatin, Glucophage and Coversyl.

After I started on the Glucophage, my glucose count improved a bit for a while. I was about 10 kilos (25 pounds) overweight, so I tried to control what I was eating. I managed to bring my weight down somewhat by reducing my intake of food. Then the weight started to come back on again.

And my glucose levels started to worsen. I decided it was time to get serious about my health.

Getting serious about my health was easier said than done. I was following the advice I had been given by medical professionals, doing all the right things according to that advice, yet still my diabetes and general health were getting steadily worse.

Was the advice I was getting wrong or seriously deficient? Perhaps I was misinterpreting it? My basic problem was ignorance.

As a consultant I had always found that the surest and easiest way to overcome ignorance is to ask questions and get answers from several sources, compare the answers and then arrive at a 'best opinion'. So I started to research diabetes mellitus (type 2 diabetes) on the internet. It was very confusing and frustrating at first, then it became fun, and finally highly illuminating.

I found out that I was not the only person searching for advice on diabetes ... many others were finding that conventional medications and diets were not stopping the progress of the disease.

I found out about the different types of diabetes and what seems to cause them. I developed some inkling as to how my bodily systems were functioning (or mal-functioning in my case), which I have described in this book.

In brief, the digestive system extracts glucose from the food you eat and releases it into the blood-stream. The blood-stream carries the glucose to your muscle cells. The glucose enters the cells and provides them with the energy they need to function.

However in order to get into the cells, insulin has to be present in the blood-stream. In type 2 diabetes, the pancreas creates and releases insulin into the bloodstream just as it does in a healthy person, and that insulin is present when the glucose is trying to enter the muscle cells.

But the insulin does not do its job of getting the glucose into the cells. This is called insulin insensitivity.

The big question was ... why is the body of a type 2 diabetic insensitive to insulin? The answer, I figured, would point to the cure.

Once I had that basic knowledge ... knew what was going wrong ... I started looking for a cure.

I did not find a cure. There isn't any.

But I did discover that I could beat diabetes ... prevent its horrendous consequences from developing.

The light dawned when I started checking statistics. I ran comparisons on the incidences of diabetes in different regions and cultures. The results were an eye-opener.

In the lesser developed world, especially in parts of Africa, where traditional plant-based diets are still the norm, diabetes is almost non-existent. However, it is growing in countries that are developing and changing to Western diets, ie, the Asian countries. In the West (Europe and North America) the disease seems to be rampant but under-reported.

It did not take much to figure out that there is something in the Western diet that triggers type 2 diabetes.

Another thing I realised is that low-carbohydrates diets ... as recommended by conventional clinics for diabetes and advisory groups such as the American Diabetes Association ... are not eaten by peoples who rarely suffer from diabetes. In fact, these people seem to eat considerably more carbohydrates (in the form of grains, noodles and starchy vegetables) than Europeans or North Americans, and treat meat as a condiment rather than an essential part of a dish.

The healthiness of the Japanese population has been well researched. The genes that allow diabetes to develop are just as common in Japanese as in Westerners. Yet, among Japanese adults who follow a traditional diet, the incidence of diabetes is only 2%. In addition ... only 1% of Japanese are clinically obese (compared to 30% of American adults) ... heart disease is rare in Japan ... some forms of cancer are also rare in that country ... and the average longevity of Japanese is better than that of Europeans or Americans.

Unfortunately for Japan and other Asian countries, such as Thailand and Vietnam, an invasion by McDonald's, KFC, and Burger King et al means grease-packed foods like meat and cheese are displacing rice and vegetables.

In Japan, in 1980, the prevalence of diabetes in all adults over the age of forty (irrespective of whether they were eating a tradition Japanese or a Western diet) was still less than 5 percent. By 1990, in just 10 years, the incidence had risen to 12 percent. Today the Japanese are busy catching up with the Americans.

It seems that the diabetes gene is like a seed – it tends not to germinate on dry (grease-free) soil. But once the Big M had started to flood the soil with processed meats and cheese, the genetic traits kicked in. That big yellow M is really a symbol of death.

So it seems that people who eat lots of carbohydrates (ie, sugar and starch) have very little diabetes. But when they begin following the Western dietary model by swopping the carbohydrates in their diet for meat and grease, they begin developing diabetes more and more.

The only possible conclusion is that high-carbohydrate diets do not cause diabetes.

Another thing that I discovered was that the unhealthy effects of the Western diet were shown up by the autopsies undertaken on the corpses of American soldiers killed during the Vietnam War. The American military carries out post-mortem examinations on its own dead as a matter of course.

Most of the more than 50,000 Americans who died in Vietnam were young male soldiers in their late teens and early twenties, and most of them would have been burger munchers. Their autopsies showed high incidences of fatty deposits in their blood and other precursors of heart disease, diabetes and kidney failure. While war stress may have played its part, the diet Uncle Sam was feeding to his boys certainly wasn't helping them.

The conclusion I came to after several weeks of research is that the problem for type 2 diabetics is not carbohydrates – the problem is how the body processes them. There is something in the Western diet, some ingredient that affects the body's ability to absorb and use carbohydrates – that prevents insulin from doing its job of getting glucose into cells.

That ingredient is fat.

I decided that eliminating fat from my diet might help my body to process carbohydrates better. I changed my diet accordingly. And it worked.

In the autumn of 2009 I was on a conventional diet for diabetics, which was:

- *Low sugar* ... no sugar in my tea or coffee, no soft drinks, no cakes, and very little jam or marmalade, and only three pieces of fruit (including 1/2 a glass of unsweetened juice) a day
- *Low fat* ... reduced bacon and sausages, grilled rather than fried meats, low-fat meats, low-fat milk and yoghurts, low-fat spreads instead of butter
- *High fibre* ... plenty of porridge, cereals and vegetables
- *Low carbohydrate* ... reduced potatoes, rice, and so on

The trick, I was told, was to divide the dinner plate into three parts – one third for vegetables, one third for protein (eg, meat or fish) and one third for carbohydrates (potatoes, pasta, rice, etc). I did so, religiously. I was also making an effort to eat less than I had been eating. In addition, I was taking 1000mg of Glucophage (metformin) a day, 500mg at breakfast and another 500mg in the evening at dinner, in order to improve my body's sensitivity to insulin.

So I was doing all the right things according to the conventional treatment for diabetes. But still my average blood glucose levels kept creeping upwards. I was keeping detailed records. When I showed these at the diabetes clinic, I was told that this was due to 'the progress of the disease', just to keep trying and to keep my eye on the condition of my feet (which were getting slightly worse every few months).

At the same time, my weight was stubbornly refusing to drop permanently – it was like a yo-yo: I'd manage to get a few pounds off and soon it would come clawing back onto my gut.

The conventional diets for diabetics were just not working for me. But the results of my research had made me feel confident enough to try something of my own devising. I felt I had the knowledge.

I decided I would eliminate all fat, as far as possible, from my diet.

My research had shown me where the fat in my diet lay. I eliminated those foods – all dairy products and most meat and fish products. My 'new' plant-focused diet was as follow:

- *No dairy products at all* ... no milk, no cheese, no yoghurts, nothing with casein (the protein found in milk which is often used in other products) in it
- *No animal fats* ... trimming off all fat from meat and fish and reducing consumption of animal products and excluding eggs entirely
- *No processed meats* ... no bacon, no rashers, no sausages, no blood puddings black or white, etc
- *Plenty of fruit* ... at least five servings a day, often more
- *Plenty of vegetables* ... all you can eat
- *Foods with low glycemic index values* ... foods that release glucose into the blood-stream slowly

I made the change suddenly and abruptly. I had researched what I could eat under a plant-focused diet and had plenty of recipes and dishes that seemed to fit the bill. I did an instant switchover in early November 2009.

Nothing happened at first. I still felt the same. My average blood glucose levels stayed the same; they seemed to have stopped going up but they did not drop either. My weight, too, remained constant.

After a week or so I was thinking of giving up. Nothing had happened. The only thing that kept me going was that I had discovered a whole new range of tastes based on vegetables that I found both intriguing and delicious. After a year off the fags (cigarettes), my taste buds had begun to sparkle.

I really began to enjoy food again. I learned a great truth … that, with the exception of mother's milk, all our tastes and habits in food are acquired.

Then it happened.

At the end of the third week, I noticed that my weight was beginning to drop. It began dropping steadily. My average glucose levels also began dropping. The drops picked up speed.

My weight was now dropping about 2kg (5lbs) a week. My energy levels picked up. I felt great. After another three weeks, I had lost 22 pounds and my weight had stabilised and my BMI reading was 23, precisely where it should be. My average blood glucose level also stabilised at a 'normal' level.

Once it began, my weight loss was so rapid that my family became worried and sent me off to see my doctor. When I showed him how I had changed my diet, he laughed and said there was nothing to worry about. The weight-loss effect of my diet was entirely to be expected.

That Christmas, I had a dietary lapse and my weight and blood glucose went up a bit. In early 2010 I went back onto my plant-focused diet. My blood glucose levels and weight returned to where I wanted them to be.

By mid-2010 I felt confident enough to reduce my Glucophage (metformin) by 50 percent. My glucose levels remained stable. In early 2011, I cut out the drug entirely. I do not seem to need a drug that makes my body more sensitive to insulin any more.

I feel that the reason I could cut out metformin is that, rather than compensating for malfunctioning insulin (which is essentially what various medications for type 2 diabetes do), the simple change in diet I undertook is helping my body's own insulin work properly again by improving the sensitivity of my body cells to insulin ... the key issue in type 2 diabetes.

That's my story.

If this book was just about my story, it would be a very short one indeed. The real reason for writing this book is to explain my understanding of type 2 diabetes and how I am managing to beat it. I feel strongly that what worked for me can work for you, for most people with type 2 diabetes.

Note that I said 'beaten', not 'cured'. There is no cure ... but this horrible disease can be beaten.

Here's what you will find in this book:

Section One ... outlines the basic information you need to understand diabetes and how it can be beaten. It covers a range of topics including the nature of the disease and how it interferes with the workings of your body, its horrendous consequences, how to monitor your diabetes, the relationship between diabetes, blood pressure, cholesterol levels and weight, and the need to deal with all these issues in order to beat your diabetes.

Section Two ... presents the information you need to make informed decisions when deciding what foods you should eat. It covers the features of diabetes-beating food ... natural (unprocessed) foods that are low in sugar, fat and salt, have plenty of fibre and low glycemic index values. Each of these attributes has a separate chapter. The section also includes a chapter on dietary supplements.

Section Three ... shows you the particular foods you should or should not eat to beat your diabetes. The section is organised into separate chapters for the various categories of food ... grains, legumes, vegetables, fruit, meat and fish, and eggs. It includes a fairly detailed look at the nutrients obtained from particular foods. It lists the foods that need to be avoided in a diabetes-beating diet. I found that, once you scratch these foods, you can eat as much as you want of the vast array of foods that are still on the menu.

Section Four ... wraps up *Beating Diabetes* up with some tips on cooking, checklists for monitoring your condition, and checklists of the foods you may eat and should not eat. It also discusses what you need to look for when you go shopping.

Note ... this book does not contain any recipes. My excuse is that the main purpose of the book is to give you the information you need to make your own cooking and eating decisions ... though perhaps the real reason for the lack of recipes is that I have not had time to sort and edit the recipes I use. In addition, the book is long enough as it is. But I will (hopefully) be creating a recipe book in the near future.

Warning

When reading this book, remember that I am not a medical doctor, I am not a scientist, and I am not a dietician or a food scientist. In fact, I am a management consultant, researcher and writer.

I have no knowledge of diabetes or any medical matters ... other than what I have found through research on the internet. All this research was 'second-hand'. I did not do any original research. All I did was read the researches of others and the conclusions they had reached.

However, my training as an accountant and auditor has endowed me with a healthy scepticism which I have brought to bear on the tasking of understanding diabetes, while twenty years of experience as a consultant has equipped me with the necessary skills to find, assess, cross-check, and filter information.

Research ... the sussing out of truth ... is a fundamental aspect of my role as a business advisor. In addition, my own health and wellbeing depends on unearthing the verifiable facts about diabetes. Indeed, my sole criterion for judging the worth of a food is the effect it will have on my health and in beating my diabetes. Thus my conclusions are likely to be unbiased.

However, you should think carefully before following my example and switching to a plant-focused diet. To be on the safe side, you should read what I say and then do your own research to confirm what I say. You should also discuss the change in your diet with a doctor or other medical advisor.

But even if my plant-based diet does not help you as much it helped me, you will still be eating good food, so it won't harm or kill you, and it's extremely unlikely it will make your diabetes worse.

And if it doesn't work, you can always switch back to a fat-soaked Western diet. But I don't think you will ... you'll find the vegetables and fruit in a plant-focused diet too delicious to give up.

To help you beat your diabetes, you can download a booklet of handy checklists and other material from www.beating-diabetes.com. The contents include:

- Checklist for monitoring diabetes
- Checklist for a diabetes-beating diet
- Conversion chart
- Fibre check
- Table of GI values
- Dietary guidelines
- Reading food labels

Find DOWNLOADS in the right-hand side-bar and click on 'Sign up and download Checklists & References'. Once you have completed the sign-up process you will receive the PDF booklet *Checklists & References* as an email attachment which you can open and save to your hard disk in the usual way.

Contents

Section One: The Fundamentals

Trying to manage diabetes is hard because if you don't, there are consequences you'll have to deal with later in life ... Bryan Adams

The purpose of this section is to give you the basic information needed to beat diabetes and related conditions.

Warning: all the information in this section was obtained through research on the internet. As such, it may not be wholly accurate or it may be that I have over-simplified the concepts. Nevertheless, this background knowledge did help me to devise the diet I am using to beat my diabetes.

1 - The Food System and Diabetes

One of the most fascinating aspects of my research was finding out how my body worked.

Up to then I had not given much thought to what is an extremely complicated, yet highly efficient, machine.

Did you ever think about what happens when you eat?

Most foods are a combination of carbohydrates, proteins and fats. A piece of meat contains mostly protein and fats. Vegetables such as potatoes contain lots of carbohydrates.

Food also contains other things such as minerals and vitamins. These are not nutrients as such, but they do help your body perform certain functions, such as aiding digestion. They act as supplements and, like food, are vital for health.

When you digest a bit of food it is broken down into the main components of food ... carbohydrates, proteins and fats. These components are then broken down further in your digestive system and are then released into to your blood-stream which delivers them around your body.

Where does your energy come from? ... from glucose.

Glucose is just a simple sugar. But, in fact, it is your body's primary source of energy.

Most glucose comes from digesting the sugar and starch in carbohydrates which you get from food such as rice, pasta, grains, breads, potatoes, fruits and some vegetables. The glucose produced by digestion in your stomach is absorbed into your bloodstream which delivers it to your body's cells.

Glucose is the fuel for your cells. Whenever you talk, walk, run, read a book, think, and so on, you are being powered by glucose ... it powers your movements, thoughts and just about everything else you do.

In order to power your cells, glucose has to get into them. It can only do this with the help of insulin.

Insulin is a hormone (a type of chemical). It is produced by your pancreas, an organ in your abdomen. The pancreas releases insulin into your bloodstream where it travels around your body and meets up with glucose on the same trip. The purpose of insulin is to enable glucose to enter your cells.

To do this, insulin attaches itself to a receptor in the surface of the cell and causes the cell membrane to allow glucose to enter the cell. The cell can then use the glucose as its fuel.

I call this the **glucose-insulin system**. It has to work properly if you are to be healthy.

If the insulin does not do its job of 'opening the cell door' for glucose, the glucose will not be able to get into the cell ... and the cell will run out of fuel.

If that happens to enough cells in your body, you will feel tired and listless ... because the cells affected will, in essence, be starving and will not have the energy that keeps your muscles active.

Diabetes is a condition in which the glucose-insulin system does not function correctly.

There are two major types of diabetes: (a) type 1 and (b) type 2.

In **type 1 diabetes** the pancreas does not produce any insulin or, at best, very little. The only way these diabetics can survive is by taking regular shots of insulin ... often several times a day ... which is why type 1 is often called *insulin-dependent diabetes*.

Type 1 diabetes is also called *childhood onset diabetes* because it usually shows up during childhood or the teenage years.

This type of diabetes cannot be cured ... a person with type 1 diabetes has to have daily injections of insulin all his or her life because their pancreas is not working properly.

This book does not deal with type 1 diabetes.

In **type 2 diabetes**, the pancreas does produce insulin which is released into the bloodstream. The problem arises at the cell door, so as to speak. When the insulin arrives at a cell it has trouble attaching itself to a receptor. So it cannot induce the cell membrane to open and allow glucose to enter the cell.

Insulin resistance is the condition in which insulin is unable to attach itself to cell receptors.

Imagine a key trying to slide into a lock in a door. If the lock is jammed ... say, with a bit of chewing gum ... the key cannot get in. There is nothing wrong with the key and nothing wrong with the lock. But before the key can get in, the lock has to be cleaned out.

One of the main reasons for insulin resistance is having cell 'doors' that are jammed with fat.

The purpose of this book is to show you how to clean out those locks of fat ... through diet and mild exercise. I did it ... so you can too!

But before we move on, there was another question that intrigued me:

Genetic influences

Why do some people develop diabetes and others, who have the same unhealthy lifestyle, manage to avoid the disease?

In my research, I discovered that diabetes seems to run in families, which means it must have a genetic basis. However the diabetes gene does not 'dictate' that something will happen but only makes it possible for diabetes to develop.

For example, if the gene that controls the colour of your eyes says that you eyes will be blue, then your eyes will be blue and there is nothing you can do about it. The same goes for the type and colour of your hair ... if your genes order wavy, brown hair for you then that's what you get.

The kinds of genes that govern diabetes are different ... they do not give orders. They merely state that if certain conditions come about then you will get diabetes, ie they predispose you to getting the disease.

If your parents were diabetic, it is likely that you inherited the genes that predispose your for type 2 diabetes. So, if you eat the same food as your parents, you are likely to develop diabetes ... but if you change your diet and lifestyle, you can probably avoid your parents' fate.

But before I show you how to do that, we'll have a quick look at the consequences of diabetes ... what happens if you do not get it under control.

These consequences are truly frightening.

Warning ... the above description of how the glucose-insulin system works is over-simplified. But it's enough to understand what's going on and how my diet can help beat type 2 diabetes.

2 - The Consequences of Diabetes

When your glucose-insulin system is not working properly ... when your insulin is unable to unlock the doors and get the glucose into your cells ... what happens?

What happens is ... a massive two-fold problem arises:

(1) Your cells are being deprived of the glucose they need to function; and

(2) You've got glucose swirling along in your bloodstream unable to do what it is supposed to do.

Depriving your cells of glucose means that you are going to be listless and unable to do all the things you do with the same energy as before. Your movements and thoughts, just about everything you do will start to slow down. You'll find that you are becoming tired more easily ... because glucose is a source of energy and your cells are being deprived of their basic food.

You may also start to lose weight because your cells are, in essence, starving ... if this happens, your arms and legs are likely to become thin and may eventually end up looking like sticks.

At the same time, the glucose in your bloodstream will have to go somewhere.

As the glucose builds up in the blood, your body wants to get rid of it ... the glucose starts to pass through the kidneys and ends up in the urine. This leads to frequent urination and a non-stop feeling of thirst.

Getting rid of the glucose also puts a strain on your kidneys ... it ends up damaging them.

Hence getting your blood glucose levels under control is vital.

But too much glucose in your bloodstream won't just damage your kidneys. It will also wreak havoc with your arteries, heart and the blood vessels of your eyes, nerves, feet and hands.

If you do not manage to control your blood glucose levels, you will surely end up with several of these awful health problems ... heart disease ... stroke ... kidney disease ... nerve damage ... neuropathy of the feet and hands ... digestive problems ... damaged eyes due to glaucoma, cataracts and retinopathy.

You are also likely to experience a variety of infections.

Heart disease

Most diabetics who do not control their blood glucose levels are killed by heart disease, one of the most common complications of diabetes.

Actually, the risk of developing heart problems depends on ... your age ... family history ... smoking habits ... weight ... cholesterol levels ... and hypertension (high blood pressure) ... as well as diabetes.

Smoking, high cholesterols levels and high blood pressure are probably the three most important of these risk factors. However, high cholesterol and blood pressure levels usually go hand-in-hand with diabetes, which increases the risks.

Stroke

A *stroke* is a rapid loss of brain function when the blood supply to the brain is interrupted. As a result of the lack of blood, the affected area of the brain is unable to function.

If you suffer a stroke, it is likely that you will be unable to move your arm or leg on one side of your body ... or, you may be unable to understand what people are saying or to speak. Your vision may also be affected. Strokes are the leading cause of disability in adults the USA and Europe, and the number two cause of death worldwide.

The risk factors for stroke include ... advancing age ... previous strokes ... hypertension (high blood pressure) ... diabetes ... high cholesterol levels ... and smoking. There's nothing you can do about the first two of these, but you can reduce all the other risks.

Kidney disease

Your kidneys are made up of millions of extremely small filtration units ... they purify your blood and send the waste products out into the urine. These tiny filtration units can be damaged by high blood pressure (hypertension), high blood glucose levels (diabetes), high cholesterol levels, and smoking.

Your kidneys are particularly sensitive to high blood pressure. At the same time, they play an important role in the regulation of blood pressure and if they have been damaged, they can lose some of their ability to keep your blood pressure down. The problem is circular ... high blood pressure damages the kidneys and damage to the kidneys can contribute to high blood pressure.

The only fix is to regulate your blood pressure and beat the effects of diabetes.

If you allow damage to your kidneys to develop, you will end up needing kidney dialysis three times a week ... a very inconvenient, extremely messy and highly uncomfortable procedure.

In the end, you'll probably need a kidney transplant.

Nerve damage

Your *nervous system* controls things such as your blood pressure, temperature, breathing, pulse rate and digestive system, as well as your ability to move, listen and talk. If you are a man, it also controls your erectile function. It consists of thousands of fibres that connect your brain and spinal cord to every part of your body.

Long-term diabetes can damage these nerve fibres ... this is called *diabetic neuropathy*. It develops when you have had high blood glucose levels for several years. This type of nerve damage is permanent. Once it's happened, you cannot improve it by controlling your diabetes better.

But you can prevent diabetic neuropathy in the first place ... by controlling your blood glucose levels through diet. And you can allay the symptoms (and prevent the damage getting worse) through a change in diet and exercise.

Surfing the internet, I discovered that researchers in California used a low-fat vegan diet and exercise (a 30-minute walk each day) on 21 persons with type 2 diabetes and neuropathy ... after two weeks the nerve symptoms had ceased entirely for 17 subjects and the remaining 4 were showing noticeable improvements.

Changing your diet, as you'll see later, is a wholly enjoyable experience. And a daily 30-minute stroll is a cinch. It's your call.

Damaged feet and hands

An early sign of diabetic neuropathy is a lack of the ability to feel vibrations in the feet, for example, from a tuning fork. The same sort of nerve damage can occur in your hands.

This nerve damage is known as *peripheral neuropathy*. It creates numbness, tingling, pain or weakness in your feet or hands. At times you'll feel as if your feet are on fire ... at other times you'll think they have been frozen solid. All this happens because the nerves that allow you to feel things or move your muscles have been damaged.

At first, peripheral neuropathy seems to be just a minor bother.

But it can be very dangerous. The reduced sensation in your feet leaves you vulnerable to injuries you do not feel. You can easily overlook a small cut or scrape.

However, because you are diabetic, these small cuts may take a long time to heal ... another consequence of diabetes. This gives them plenty of time to become infected. And, if these infections fester, your foot may need to be amputated.

Diabetes is a common cause of amputations of the feet and lower limbs.

Thus it is vital that you should have your feet examined by your doctor at least once a year. He or she will check for sensitivity by tickling your feet with thread and use a tuning fork to see if you can feel vibrations, as well as looking for signs of damage to the skin.

If you do have neuropathy, you should check your feet daily for signs of injury or infection. Any injuries should be treated without delay. Always wear shoes as, having lost some feeling in your feet, you may not know if you step on something sharp. To avoid blisters use shoes that fit properly. In the house, use slippers with strong rims on the sole to avoid banging your foot against furniture. You should also keep your nails trimmed neatly, but do not shorten them more than the ends of your toes.

Digestive problems
Having diabetes increases your risk of getting stomach problems, such as *gastroparesis* in which the vagus nerve that controls the muscles of the stomach and intestines is damaged and the movement of food through the digestive process is interrupted.

If you have gastroparesis, the length of time it takes for you to digest food will be unpredictable, making it very difficult to monitor your blood glucose and control the effects diabetes is having on your heart, kidneys, nerves, feet and hands, and eyes.

Gastroparesis has extremely unpleasant consequences. You may suffer from malnutrition due to the vomiting brought on by the condition. Because you will be deficient in calories, you will probably suffer severe fatigue and weight loss. It can get worse. You could end up with solid masses of undigested food in your stomach which will block your intestines. You also have a pretty good chance of getting a bacterial infection due to the undigested food and high glucose levels.

Years of high blood glucose levels will lead to gastroparesis. The best thing to do is to prevent it by gaining control of your blood glucose levels before the condition starts developing.

Eye damage

Your eye is a complex optical system which collects light, regulates its intensity through a diaphragm (the pupil), focuses it through an adjustable assembly of lenses to form an image, converts the image into electrical signals (in the retina at the back of the eye), and transmits these signals through neural pathways that connect the eye, via the optic nerves, to the visual cortex and other areas in the brain.

Your eyes also have photosensitive ganglion cells in their retinas. These do not form images. Instead they automatically adjust the size of your pupils to cope with the intensity of the light and regulate your body clock in accordance with the light.

This amazing system allows you to perceive depth and distinguish colours, and to feel sleepy when it gets dark.

Your eyes contain thousands of *capillaries*, minute hair-like blood vessels with very thin walls. Their tiny size and the thinness of their walls mean that they are very fragile. These tiny blood vessels are especially sensitive to glucose in the blood. They can be damaged by persistently high blood glucose levels and high blood pressure.

Indeed, if you are diabetic, several parts of the eye are highly susceptible to damage, and you can develop three different diseases: glaucoma, cataracts and retinopathy.

Protecting your eyes means keeping your blood glucose, blood pressure and cholesterol levels under control. Only a diet that reduces your glucose and blood pressure levels, and helps to clean out your arteries, will be kind to the tiny blood vessels in your eyes.

Researchers have discovered the some of the changes in the eyes due to diabetes, such as exudates in the retina, start to improve when a person switches to a plant-focused, minimal-fat diet.

As well as switching to a suitable diet, you should get an examination and advice from an eye specialist at least once a year … and whenever you notice any changes in your vision.

Glaucoma

If you have glaucoma your vision will have deteriorated due to damage to your optic nerve caused by pressure within the eye or a weakness in the optic nerve, or both.

What happens is that pressure builds up in the anterior chamber (the front of the eye) which pinches the tiny blood vessels in the retina. This damages both the retina and the optic nerve.

If glaucoma is discovered early, treatment can be effective. Because it can begin without symptoms, you can only catch it in time if you have your eyes examined by an ophthalmologist (eye doctor) at least once a year. If left untreated, glaucoma can make you blind.

Both high blood pressure and high glucose levels increase the risk of getting glaucoma. The best defence against its development is to keep these under control.

Cataracts

Cataracts are a painless clouding of the lens of the eye. These generally develop over a long period of time, causing eyesight to gradually get worse.

If you are starting to develop cataracts, you may notice … difficulty with your distance vision … blurred or double vision … a halo effect around lights … excessive glare in bright sunlight … or too much glare while driving at night.

If you experience any of these symptoms, you should have your eyes checked promptly.

The older you are, the more likely you are to develop cataracts, and avoiding age-related cataracts is probably impossible. Those with a family history of cataracts are most likely to develop the disease.

However, cataracts can also be caused by … diabetes … high blood pressure … smoking … alcohol … exposure to harsh sunlight … and the long-term use of steroid medicines. In addition, injuries to the eye and other eye problems can lead to cataracts.

You can retard the development of cataracts by avoiding … tobacco … fatty foods … alcohol … and dairy products … and by protecting your eyes from harsh sunlight.

Research has shown that people who avoid fats have less risk of cataracts.

The risk is also reduced by about 10% for non-drinkers … just two drinks a week is related to increased risk.

Those who avoid dairy products also have a significantly lower risk of developing cataracts. This is because the lactose (sugar) in milk releases galactose, a simple sugar, during digestion. Galactose can enter the lens of your eye and damage its tiny blood vessels.

Generally speaking, foods rich in vitamins C and E help prevent cataracts. Particular foods may also help. For example, lutein and zeaxanthin, antioxidants found in green leafy vegetables, protect the lens.

Retinopathy

Your retinas consist of millions of tiny nerves that pick up images, convert them into electrical signals and send them to the brain. These tiny nerves can be damaged by high blood glucose, high blood pressure and high concentrations of cholesterol. This damage is known as *retinopathy*.

Retinopathy does not have any symptoms when it starts. Therefore it is essential to have your eyes checked regularly ... at least once a year.

The changes caused by retinopathy cannot be detected by an ordinary eye examination using an ophthalmoscope (which a doctor would ordinarily use) or by a regular sight-test (an optometric exam) by an optician. So, you should be examined by an ophthalmologist, who will dilate your eyes so that he can see into the retina at the back of the eye.

To avoid the damage caused by retinopathy you need to maintain the correct levels for you blood glucose, cholesterol and blood pressure.

Infections

Diabetes affects your immune system and reduces your body's ability to fight infection. At the same time, high blood glucose leads to high levels of sugar in the tissues of your body.

Your weaker immunity and the presence of sugar enable bacteria and fungi to grow and infections to develop more quickly. These infections can affect your bladder, kidneys, vagina, gums, feet and skin. It is therefore vital that you control your blood glucose levels.

About one-third of people who are diabetic will get a skin infection related to their disease at some time in their lives. Fortunately, most of these skin conditions can be treated successfully.

However if you have type 2 diabetes and do not care for your skin properly, a minor skin condition can turn into a serious problem with severe consequences. You should examine your skin, especially your feet and legs, daily for any signs of infection.

For diabetics, the early treatment of all infections is vital to prevent more serious complications.

Other problems

Diabetes brings on a host of other problems, such as erectile dysfunction and dental problems.

An overview

The outlook, if you do not take steps to beat your diabetes, is extremely grim... it ranges from heart attacks through disabilities, dialysis, transplants, infections, amputation, blindness, to death.

These horrible consequences are not caused solely by diabetes. Excess blood pressure, high levels of cholesterol, smoking and being overweight also play their part in your destruction. In addition, alcohol, fatty foods and dairy products make a contribution.

It is obvious that you must control not just your diabetes but also ... your blood pressure ... cholesterol levels ... and give up smoking. If I am managing to do so, so can you.

Becoming insulin dependent

When type 2 diabetes begins to affect you ... when your body starts becoming insulin insensitive ... the levels of glucose in your blood will be rising but will still be quite low.

If you fail to control your blood glucose levels, ie fail to unblock the fat-jammed locks of your muscle cells, your pancreas will sense all the glucose swirling around in your bloodstream and will create more and more insulin.

Eventually your pancreas will realise that the insulin it is producing is not being used. It will reduce the production of insulin severely or even shut it down. Should this happen, you will need regular injections of insulin ... just like a type 1 diabetic who is insulin dependent.

Injecting insulin is a messy affair and gauging the amounts required is difficult. It is best to avoid having to do so by taking control of your diabetes.

3 - Monitoring Diabetes

As I mentioned at the start of this book, it was ridges I had noticed on the back of my tongue that led to my diagnosis of diabetes. I was scared I had cancer of the mouth or throat.

The doctor recognized them immediately for what they were ... signs that I had diabetes. She sent me to the leading diabetes unit in the Gulf to have the diagnosis confirmed.

There are a variety of symptoms a person may have that indicate diabetes. The three main ones are: ... a need to urinate frequently (*polyuria*) ... increased thirst and fluid intake (*polydipsia*), and ... increased appetite (*polyphagia*).

These symptoms are caused by the effect of diabetes on the body. Once the level of glucose in the blood has become too high, it starts to pass through your kidneys and ends up in your urine.

To get through your kidneys, the glucose needs plenty of water ... hence you need to pass water often. And naturally, losing all that fluid makes you thirsty. You probably feel extra hungry because your cells are not getting the food (glucose) they need.

Other symptoms of diabetes, which I only found out about when I started researching the matter seriously, include ... blurred vision ... cuts or sores that take a long time to heal ... itching skin or yeast infections ... dry mouth ... and pain in the feet or legs.

Strangely, the only reason I went to the doctor was the ridges on the back of my tongue. I did not find these mentioned as a symptom anywhere during my research. In other words, I was developing diabetes without experiencing any of the normally-expected symptoms. Talk about a silent killer!

For this reason I feel, strongly, that everyone who is getting on in age ... already on the upside of 40 ... should be tested for diabetes on a regular basis, say once a year.

Getting tested

Anyway, to pick up the story, I went to the diabetes clinic having fasted overnight. A sample of my blood was taken and I was told to go home, eat my normal breakfast and come back two hours later. I did. They took my blood again. I had the results within a few minutes. I was borderline diabetic.

The clinic asked me to do a more formal test. This time I fasted for a full 12 hours overnight before going to the clinic in the morning. They took my blood and determined the pre-prandial (before eating) level of glucose in my blood.

Then I had a glucose tolerance test. I was given a glass of sugary fluid to drink, a syrup containing 75gm of glucose and nothing else (except water). I drank this down and waited.

After two hours my blood was taken again to measure the post-prandial (after eating) blood glucose level, and the diagnosis was confirmed ... prediabetes.

These tests are based on how your body responds when you eat some food. Digestion begins immediately. The digestive process breaks down the food and glucose begins to be released into your bloodstream. The level of glucose in your blood begins to rise, which is normal and expected.

After a while the level reaches a peak and then begins to drop off as the glucose gets into your cells (provided you don't have diabetes). In a healthy person, the level of blood glucose will have dropped back down to about its normal level after two hours or so (depending on the quantity of food taken).

The simple laboratory tests I underwent measured the amount of glucose in my blood both before and two hours after eating. The results showed whether I had excess glucose in my blood both before and after food.

But how is glucose in the blood measured?

Measuring glucose
Throughout most of the world, the amount of glucose in your blood is measured in millimoles per litre (mmol/l) in accordance with the Système International d'Unités (SI units).

The exceptions are the USA, Liberia and Myanmar where the glucose is measured in milligrams per decilitre (mg/dl), ie one-thousandths of a gram in a tenth of a litre.

In case you're wondering – a *millimole* is one thousandth of a mole. A *mole* is the amount of a substance that contains as many molecules as the number of atoms in 12 grams of carbon-12.

If you don't understand what this means, don't worry. All you need to realise is that a millimole is a very accurate measurement of an extremely tiny amount of something ... at the level of the molecule. Essentially the mmol/l figures tells you how many molecules of glucose (or cholesterol, or any other substance such as triglycerides), divided by a thousand, there are in a litre of your blood.

The SI units are much more accurate than the American system. This is because the SI units measure the number of molecules of a substance in the blood, while the American system only considers the weight of that substance.

The conversion factor for blood glucose measurements is 18 ... to convert from mmol/l to mg/dl you multiply the mmol/l figure by 18. To convert from the American to the SI units, you divide by 18. For example, 5.6 mmol/l = 100.8 mg/dl.

As the mass of a mole varies with the molecular weight of the substance being analysed, converting between the American and SI units requires differing conversion factors depending on the substance being measured. In other words, the conversion factor for glucose in blood will not be the same as the conversion factor for cholesterol or triglycerides.

There are conversion charts in *Checklists & References* which you can find at www.beating-diabetes.com under DOWNLOADS.

Levels of blood glucose

What are the correct levels for the glucose in your blood?

The normal glucose level for a healthy (non-diabetic) person is:
- less than 5.6mmol/l (100mg/l) ... after fasting for 8 hours
- less than 7.8 mmol/l (140 mg/l) ... after a two-hour glucose tolerance test (in which a syrup made up of water and 75gms of glucose taken on a fasting stomach)

You will be clinically diagnosed as having diabetes if you blood glucose level is:
- 7.0 mmol/l (126 mg/dl) or more ... after fasting for 8 hours
- 11.1mmol/l (200 mg/dl) or more ... after a two-hour glucose tolerance test
- 11.1mmol/l (200 mg/dl) or more ... at any time and whether or not you have been fasting

If your blood glucose levels are above the normal limits but not high enough to warrant a diagnosis of diabetes, you will be diagnosed as having impaired glucose tolerance or pre-diabetes.

When I was first tested in Kuwait, my blood glucose levels were around 6.2mmol/l (111.6mg/dl) both pre- and post-prandial.

Pre-diabetes ... impaired glucose tolerance ... means that you are on your way to developing diabetes and need to take suitable changes to your diet and lifestyle to prevent the disease from developing.

I failed to take those precautions.

Monitoring and recording

It seems obvious but, to know whether any steps you are taking to control your diabetes are being effective, you need to track your blood glucose levels. Doing so is easy using a small portable tester.

The little machine comes with a 'pricker' and disposable lancets for making a tiny pin hole in the finger, and disposable 'test strips' which are inserted into the tester each time you do a check.

To check your blood, you just insert a test strip into the machine, prick your finger, dip the end of the test strip into the little bubble of blood that bubbles up through the tiny hole in your finger ... and in a few seconds the tester will show the level of the glucose in your blood in big bold numbers.

To ensure that there is nothing on your skin which might interfere with an accurate reading, you should wash your hands ... especially the fingers from which you will be taking blood ... before you use the lancet.

This is particularly necessary if you have been handling fruit or reading a newspaper. The sugars in fruit skins and in newsprint can cause readings to be high.

Do not use alcohol rubs or swabs to clean your fingers before testing. The alcohol can fix sugars and other carbon-based chemicals to the skin. But you should, as a precaution, wipe the prick hole in your finger with alcohol after testing to prevent infection.

Some people check their glucose levels only now-and-then. I like to do it four times a day ... on arising in the morning and two hours after each main meal, ie, breakfast, lunch and dinner.

Some doctors recommend that you check your blood immediately before you eat and then two hours after you finish. This gives you a before-and-after view of your blood glucose levels. It seems a good idea to me ... but it's a bit fiddly in practice.

However often you check your blood, it is important that you record the readings ... otherwise you won't be able to see how well you are controlling your blood glucose levels over time.

To record each reading, I use MS Excel, a computer spreadsheet program, as it makes it easy to calculate the overall average for the week and the week's averages for the various times of the day when I check my blood. The summarised data enables me to see the trends in my glucose levels.

Your blood glucose readings taken two hours after each meal will vary depending on what and how much you have eaten and what you did in the intervening two hours. For this reason, I like to record a summary of the food I have eaten as well.

To ensure I don't forget to check my blood two hours after a meal, I use the reminder function in my mobile ... this works fine as long as I remember to put in the reminder when I've finished my meal!

It's often difficult to check your blood glucose four to eight times a day ... every day. However, as long as you check your blood on average twice a day at varying times you will be building up a good record of your blood glucose levels. After a few weeks you will easily be able to see whether the efforts you are making to control your glucose levels are paying off or not.

Trends in glucose levels
Watching the trends is crucial to controlling your blood glucose levels.

Glucose levels will bounce around a bit from day to day. These differences are not always related to the food you eat. They can be due to more or less exercise, work, travel, and so on. An illness, flu or other infection, or other injury can boost glucose levels. Stress will also increase levels dramatically. Ups and downs are normal. So don't fret. Wait for the overall trends to show up.

Your blood glucose level can sometimes be higher in the morning than it was just before going to bed at night. This is normal. However I found it worrying until I discovered the simple explanation.

Glucose is vital for the functioning of the body, especially the brain. The body constantly monitors and alters the amount of glucose in the bloodstream. It increases the level when it gets too low.

In the early hours of the morning the level can get too low. When this happens, hormones cause the liver to release glucose into the blood-stream. This can raise blood glucose levels significantly.

The body's system for controlling blood glucose levels is a bit imprecise ... it doesn't take into account the fact that you are sleeping and don't need extra energy.

Blood sugar levels are a bit like the stock-market ... they fluctuate up and down all the time, hour by hour and day by day. It's the overall trend that is important ... is the average increasing gradually or decreasing over time?

As well as tracking your average levels of blood glucose on a daily and weekly basis, there is another, excellent, way to find out how well you are controlling your diabetes.

Haemoglobin A1c

Haemoglobin A1c (HbA1C) is the principal gauge of blood glucose control ... of how well you are controlling your diabetes. In comparison, blood glucose testing only indicates how you are doing at the time you take the test.

Haemoglobin (spelt *hemoglobin* in the USA) is the pigment that gives the colour to your red blood cells. If you have had a lot of glucose in your blood, plenty of it will have gotten into your red blood cells and will have stuck to your haemoglobin. If you have not had much glucose in your blood, your haemoglobin will have much less glucose stuck to it.

The A1c test measures how much glucose has stuck to haemoglobin. It is measured in two different ways: (a) as a percentage (eg, 7%) or (b) as millimoles per mol (ie, as thousandths of moles per mole, eg 53 mmol/mol). The latter is the more accurate measure.

The relationship between the two forms of measurement is not wholly linear.

To convert the percent measure to mmol/mol, you deduct 2.15 from the percent figure and multiply the result by 10.929. For example, 6% = (6.0-2.15) x 10.929 = 42 mmol/mol.

To convert mmol/mol to percent, you divide the mmol/mol figure by 10.929 and add 2.15 to the result. For example, 75mmol/mol = (75/10.929) + 2.15 = 9%.

There is a conversion chart for the two forms of measurement in *Checklists & References* which you can find at www.beating-diabetes.com under DOWNLOADS.

More millimoles per mole or a higher percentage means that more glucose is attached to your haemoglobin than for lower numbers.

Red blood cells have a life span of three to four months ... so the A1c test indicates how well your blood glucose has been controlled over the previous three months or so.

Thus it is best to check your HbA1c levels every three months or, at least, every six months. Once a year is not enough to keep tabs on what's happening with your glucose levels.

Effects of high HbA1c levels

A few years ago, the recommendation was that persons with diabetes get their HbA1c values below 53mmol/mol (7%). Based on recent research, many experts are now recommending target levels of 48mmol/mol (6.5%) or lower.

The *Prospective Diabetes Study* in the UK has shown that a 1% drop in HbA1c levels for people with type-2 diabetes lowers the risk of eye or kidney problems by about 37% ... a clear indication that lower values cut the risk of diabetic complications.

The higher the HbA1c level, the greater is the risk of circulatory problems. Keeping HbA1c levels low has been found to be important for the health of your eyes, kidneys and nerves in particular. Studies have found that people who keep their HbA1c levels low encounter fewer heart problems as they age.

Reducing HbA1c levels

Large-scale research has shown that, on average ... the diet recommended by the American Diabetes Association reduces HbA1c levels by 0.4% ... using metformin (Glucophage), a diabetes medicine, reduces HbA1c levels by 0.6%, and ... a vegan diet (no meat or dairy products) reduces HbA1c levels by 1.2%.

Thus, a typical oral medication for diabetes brings HbA1c levels down by just over half a percent ... while a vegan diet has about twice the effect of a standard medication ... and a vegan diet has three times the effect the conventional diet recommended for diabetics.

The effect of a vegan diet will depend on a variety of factors ... your HbA1c level when you start the diet ... how well you stick to the diet ... how much weight you lose ... how much exercising you do ... and your genes (which you inherit and cannot change).

Personally, I managed to bring my HbA1c levels down significantly (to just over 42mmol/mol or 6%) without resorting to a wholly vegan diet. I don't eat any dairy products (milk, cheese, etc) or eggs but still eat a little meat (with all the fat removed) so I am close to a vegan diet.

Exercising has also been found to reduce HbA1c levels. But the research I perused was not referring to strenuous exercise. Exercise in this context was just a minimum of four hours of walking, cycling or light gardening a week, not a heavy load.

A long-term tracking study (over nearly two decades) found that persons with type-2 diabetes who did just four hours of this type of exercise a week had a 40% lower risk of heart disease than sedentary diabetics. These people also cut their risk of stroke.

Thus, exercise is obviously important. But its benefits are not as marked as the effects of a change to a healthy diet ... which is what I have concentrated on, with plenty of success.

Regular testing

It is vital that you have your HbA1c levels tested three times a year, ie every four months (the life-cycle of your red blood cells). This is the only sure-fire way to know whether your efforts to control you blood glucose levels and beat your diabetes are working.

At the same time you must continue to check your blood glucose levels several times a day. If you don't, you are likely to let your diet slip, which is what happened initially in my case.

So stay on track with ... daily checks, and ... four monthly confirmations.

The risk of hypoglycaemia

Hypoglycaemia is a fall in blood glucose to dangerously low levels, ie, below 3.9mmol/l (70mg/dl).

The bad news about hypoglycaemia (for anyone, even if you are healthy) is that there is a risk that you will fall unconscious. The good news (for a diabetic) is that hypoglycaemia is a sign that your body is regaining its insulin sensitivity.

The symptoms of hypoglycaemia include ... sweating ... shaking ... hunger ... anxiety ... weakness ... a rapid heartbeat ... dizziness or light-headedness ... sleepiness or confusion ... and difficulty speaking.

Hypoglycaemia can be brought on by vigorous exercise. It can also occur during the night ... indeed any time you have used up a lot of energy or have not eaten for a long time.

As far as I was able to find out, hypoglycaemia is unlikely if you are not taking any medications for diabetes or are only being treated with Glucophage (metformin) or thiazolidinediones such as Actos (pioglitazone) or Avandia (rosiglitazone) … provided you are taking regular meals or snacks.

However I feel that, if you are taking medication for your diabetes and are also starting a new diet (with or without additional exercise), you should be aware of the possibility of experiencing hypoglycaemia. Here's some advice I found on the internet.

If you are susceptible to hypoglycaemia, you should carry glucose tablets plus your tester. If you do experience the symptoms of hypoglycaemia, you should check your blood and if it is below 3.9mmol/l (70mg/dl), you should ingest some sugar by taking … 15gms of glucose tablets, or … 1/2 a glass of fruit juice, or … 1/2 a glass of any soft drink except a diet drink (you want the sugar!), or … half-a-dozen pieces of sucky sweets (hard candy), or … 1 or 2 teaspoons of sugar.

You should retest your glucose level after 15 minutes. If the level is still below 3.9mmol/l, take more sugar … and contact your doctor immediately.

4 - Three-in-one: Metabolic Syndrome

Most of us with type 2 diabetes have, in addition to problems with the amount of glucose in our blood, difficulties with the levels of our blood pressure, cholesterol and triglycerides.

In other words, we have the so-called three-in-one or metabolic syndrome.

The term *metabolic* refers to the biochemical processes that take place in your body when it is functioning normally. A *syndrome* is a set of several distinct symptoms that are regularly found together in a particular grouping. There are numerous medical syndromes.

Metabolic syndrome is a cluster of disorders concerning certain biochemical processes ... high blood glucose levels, increased blood pressure, abnormal cholesterol levels, or excess body fat around the waist ... that very often occur at the same time in your body.

You have metabolic syndrome if you have any three of the following symptoms:

(a) your blood glucose after fasting of is 5.6mmol/L (100mg/dL) or more;
(b) your blood pressure is 130/85mm Hg or more;
(c) your triglycerides levels are 1.7 mmol/L (150 mg/dL) or more and your HDL ('good') cholesterol levels are less than 1.04 mmol/L (40 mg/dL) if you are a man or 1.3 mmol/L (50 mg/dL) if you are a woman; or
(d) the circumference of your waist is 102cm (40ins) or more if you are a man and 89 cm (35ins) or more if you are a woman.

But these limits can vary depending on your race.

It seems that metabolic syndrome arises before you become diabetic, and it increases your chances of developing diabetes and heart disease or of suffering a stroke. If you have one component of the syndrome, you are likely to have the others.

And the more components you have, the greater the risks to your health. Indeed, a person who has metabolic syndrome is twice as likely to develop heart disease and five times as likely to develop diabetes as someone who doesn't have the syndrome.

The syndrome includes several symptoms that have different causes. However it does seem to be linked to your body's metabolism, especially to insulin resistance. Diabetes is not the only medical condition caused by insulin resistance.

Increased insulin in your blood can interfere with the functioning of your kidneys and lead to higher blood pressure. Increased insulin can also raise the levels of your triglycerides and other blood fats. Insulin resistance is closely linked to being overweight and obese.

The syndrome can be due to a variety of causes that act together. You can control some of these causes, such as an inactive lifestyle, a poor diet and being overweight or obese.

The causes you cannot control include getting older, your genetics (certain races are more prone to insulin resistance and metabolic syndrome than others), and your family history.

Metabolic syndrome affects between 20 and 25 percent of the populations in Western countries. In addition, about 85 percent of people who have type 2 diabetes also have metabolic syndrome.

So the chances are very high that, as a type 2 diabetic, you have problems with the other components of metabolic syndrome. Thus, in order to beat your diabetes, you have to control your blood pressure, cholesterol and triglycerides, and not just your blood glucose levels.

The good news is that the diet I follow, along with a modicum of exercise, will probably be effective in controlling your hypertension (abnormally high blood pressure) and cholesterol and triglyceride levels.

5 - Controlling Blood Pressure

Blood pressure is the force against the walls of your arteries as your heart pumps blood through your body. *Hypertension* refers to blood pressure that is higher than it should be. Having hypertension or high blood pressure usually goes hand-in-hand with diabetes.

One of the problems with hypertension is that it hardly ever causes symptoms until your condition becomes severe. This means that if you don't have your blood pressure checked regularly you may not notice that you have hypertension until you begin to get heart disease or have a stroke.

I first experienced high blood pressure nearly a decade before I was diagnosed with diabetes, in Jordan after I managed to get out of Iraq-Kuwait in late 1990.

A Palestinian doctor in Jordan kindly gave me some medicine to reduce the tension. At the time I assumed, as did that good doctor, that it was just a temporary problem brought on by the stress of being one of Saddam's Guestages and travelling around Kuwait and Iraq under war conditions.

When your blood pressure goes really high, you get a headache and have a feeling that your head is very heavy, too heavy for your body. Your thinking slows down, you find it hard to concentrate and you get mildly confused. Your whole body seems tense, yet at the same time you feel really sleepy. That was my experience when I was in Jordan and why I called for a doctor.

These weird feelings abate as your blood pressure comes down. You only get them when your blood pressure is really high. Normally, when your blood pressure is moderately high, you don't notice it ... therein lies the danger.

Once I was out of Iraq my blood pressure reverted to normal. Then, a year or so later, it began to increase again and, by the time I was diagnosed with diabetes I'd been on medication for my blood pressure for seven or eight years.

First I was put on 50mg of Tenoretic a day. Tenoretic contains a medicine that causes the heart to beat slower and with less force. It also contains a diuretic which helps the kidneys to remove water from the blood into the urine, a trick that reduces the volume of blood circulating in the body and so reduces blood pressure.

However, my blood pressure was gradually getting worse. A year or so later my dosage was increased to 100mg a day and I continued to take 100mg of Tenoretic daily for several years.

One day I felt really weirdly light-headed and unable to concentrate. I went to my local government clinic in Kuwait, where I found out that my blood pressure was abnormally low. I was told that if it dropped any more I'd likely go into a coma.

I stopped taking my Tenoretic and in a day or so I felt fine. I went back to my doctor and found that my blood pressure was now normal. My hypertension had been cured!

Unfortunately, this happy state of affairs only lasted for about six months. My blood pressure began to creep up again. A year later I was back on the medicines ... this time a daily dose of 50mg of Tenormin, which is similar to Tenoretic except that it does not contain a diuretic.

By this time I had been diagnosed with diabetes. At the time I knew little about either diabetes or blood pressure. I just followed doctor's orders and took my blood-pressure medicine regularly and more or less followed the advice I received about my diabetes.

Still my blood pressure tended to fluctuate. It wasn't until I began following the diet I devised to deal with my diabetes that my blood pressure became stable and within the correct levels. Today I'm getting readings of 115/75mmHg consistently.

Until I began researching diabetes I knew little about how the body's blood circulation system works ... about what causes abnormal blood pressure ... and the serious dangers, such as heart disease, aneurisms, eye and kidney damage, and so on, that continuously high blood pressure threatens.

As a type 2 diabetic, there is an 85% chance that you also have issues with your blood pressure.

Blood circulation system

Your body has an ingenious system for delivering oxygen from your lungs and nutrients from your digestive system around your body ... the cardiovascular system.

Your heart is essentially a pump that forces blood through your body. The heart pumps blood through the arteries out to your muscles and other organs where it delivers oxygen and nutrients. The blood then returns to your heart via your veins.

Pulmonary circulation is the portion of the cardiovascular system that carries blood from your lungs, where the blood has been loaded up with oxygen, to your heart.

The *systemic circulation* carries the oxygenated blood from your heart around your body. On its way, this blood picks up nutrients released by your digestive system and delivers them, along with the oxygen, to your body cells.

Your blood also picks up other materials, such as waste, and delivers them to where they need to go. Unused glucose, for example, is delivered to the kidneys whence it passes into the urine.

This delivery system then returns the blood, which no longer carries much oxygen, back to the heart. Once the blood is back in the heart, the pulmonary circulation carries that blood back to the lungs, where the oxygen is replenished and the delivery cycle begins again.

Blood pressure

Your heart, like any pump, works by creating pressure. It is continuously expanding and contracting, which creates an on-off cycle of pressure on the blood.

Blood pressure is the pressure the circulating blood exerts on the walls of the blood vessels or tubes through which it is travelling. Your blood pressure (BP) varies rhythmically with each beat of your heart.

The *maximum (or systolic) pressure* of your blood is created when you heart beats. At the end of the pause between each beat, the pressure is at a minimum (known as the *diastolic pressure*). This on-off cycle of beats never stops (until you die).

The pressure the circulating blood exerts on the walls of the blood vessels depends on three main factors: (i) how forcefully your heart is pumping, (ii) how relaxed or wide your arteries are, and (iii) where the blood is in your body.

Like any tube, your blood vessels resist the flow of blood, and the pressure drops a bit as your blood moves away from your heart along the arteries. The pressure drops more rapidly once the blood has reached your arterioles (tiny blood vessels or tubes that branch out from the main arteries). It continues to go down as your blood moves through the capillaries (the smallest blood vessels) and then along the veins back to the heart.

This is why your blood pressure is nearly always measured at the main artery in your upper arm ... measuring it at other places on the body would give inconsistent or non-standard readings.

As well as these three main factors ... the force of your heartbeat, the resistance of your blood vessels, and its location in your body ... your blood pressure is also influenced by gravity, the valves in your veins and the contraction of your muscles as you do things. This last factor is the reason why you need to be relaxed and at rest when your blood pressure is being measured.

And, as I discovered, blood pressure is also influenced by many external factors such as ... your age ... stress ... the food you eat ... diseases ... drugs (both medical and recreational) ... and exercise.

Measuring blood pressure
Your blood pressure can be normal, too high or too low.

When the pressure in your arteries (arterial pressure) is abnormally high you have *hypertension*, which simple means that your blood is being forced through your arteries under too much pressure.

You have *hypotension* when the opposite occurs, ie your blood pressure is abnormally low.

The strength of your blood pressure is expressed as the systolic (maximum) pressure over the diastolic (minimum) pressure for each beat of your heart; eg, 120/80mmHg.

Hg is the symbol for mercury. The unit of measurement, mmHg, refers to the pressure needed to keep a column of liquid mercury at a certain height in a sealed tube. For example, 5mmHg is the pressure needed to maintain a column of mercury at a height of 5 millimetres.

Apparently it is not considered a very accurate measurement, as I found out in my research, but it is what is used.

Normal blood pressure is a pressure of less than 120/80 mmHg.

According to the American Heart Association (AHA), there are four stages hypertension ... Pre-hypertension (120/80 to 139/89 mmHg) ... Stage 1 hypertension (140/90 to 159/99 mmHg) ... Stage 2 hypertension (160/100 to 179/109 mmHg), and ... Crisis hypertension (more than 180/110 mmHg).

The problem with the AHA view is that it is based on average readings for adults aged over 18 in the population as a whole. I could not find out whether this 'average' excluded those with hypertension.

Given that the population of the USA is known to have poor health on average, I feel that the AHA figures are a bit optimistic, ie, they are a bit higher than would be appropriate for a healthy person.

A study I discovered tested 100 adults (admittedly a small sample) with no history of hypertension. Their average blood pressure was 112/64mmHg. I would consider these to be the values we should aim to achieve and maintain in order to safeguard our health.

The risk of cardiovascular disease (ie, problems relating to the heart and blood vessels) increases progressively when BP readings are above 115/75 mmHg. I found clinical trials showing that people who maintain their blood pressures below this level have much better long-term cardiovascular health. My personal aim is to get my BP down to 112/64mmHg, with 115/75 mmHg as an upper limit.

How the body regulates blood pressure

What surprised me in my research is that the way in which the body regulates its blood pressure is not yet fully understood by medical scientists.

What happens is that sensors (called *baroreceptors*) located in the blood vessels detect changes in the pressure in the arteries and send signals to the brain. The brain reacts and adjusts the blood pressure by altering the force and speed of the heart's contractions.

The kidneys also have a role to play. A system, called the Renin-angiotensin system, enables the kidneys to compensate for any loss in the volume of blood or a drop in pressure by activating angiotensin II, which is an internal vasoconstrictor. A *vasoconstrictor* contracts the wall of a blood vessel, which makes the blood vessel narrower and thus increases blood pressure within that tube.

But, if your body is capable of regulating your blood pressure, what causes high blood pressure? The short answer is ... medical scientists don't know.

For more than 90% of people with high blood pressure, the cause is not known. For the remaining 10%, the underlying cause can range from chronic kidney disease through diseases in the arteries supplying the kidneys to chronic abuse of alcohol, hormonal disturbances and endocrine tumours.

What influences blood pressure?

Your blood pressure is influenced by four factors: (i) your cardiac output, (ii) the resistance of your blood vessels, (iii) the volume of blood, and (iv) its viscosity (thickness).

(i) Your *cardiac output* is the amount and speed of the blood being pumped by your heart. It is the *stroke volume* (the amount of blood pumped out of your heart with each beat) multiplied by the *heart rate* (the speed at which your heart is beating).

If either your stroke volume or heart rate increases, while the other remains as it is, your blood pressure will go up. Vice versa, if one of them decreases, your blood pressure will drop.

(ii) The *resistance* of your blood vessels depends on the width of those tubes, on their length, and on the smoothness of the walls inside the vessels.

The larger the tubes, the easier it is for blood to flow and the resistance will be less. The longer their length, the more the effort needed to push the blood, and the resistance will be higher.

Bumps on the walls inside the blood vessels will create resistance to the flow of blood. For most of us, unfortunately, the smoothness of the walls is reduced by the build-up of fatty deposits (plaques), mainly due to the cholesterol in our diets.

The resistance of your blood vessels can be changed by using medications to increase or decrease their size. *Vasodilators*, such as nitro-glycerine, increase the size of tubes and decrease the pressure in the arteries. *Vasoconstrictors* reduce the size of your blood vessels and so increase your BP.

(iii) The *volume of blood* is the amount of blood you have in you. If the volume of your blood increases, your cardiac output will also and your blood pressure will go up.

There is a relationship between the amount of salt in your food and increased blood volume which is why taking a lot of salt in your food tends to increase your BP.

(iv) The *viscosity* or thickness of your blood also affects your BP. If your blood gets thicker, your BP will go up as it takes more effort to move it along.

Some medical conditions can change the viscosity of your blood, eg anaemia.

Your blood pressure is never static. The systolic and diastolic blood pressures in your arteries are constantly varying … from one heartbeat to another … and throughout the day. Your BP also changes in response to stress, your diet, drugs, disease, exercise, and momentarily when you stand up. These variations can be quite large.

Most people who have hypertension do not usually show any symptoms … a main reason why high blood pressure is seldom detected unless you are having a routine medical examination or are being checked for some other condition, such as diabetes.

However, if you have severe hypertension, you will experience headaches, sleepiness, confusion, and, if you blood pressure is extremely high, you could fall into a coma.

Consequences of high blood pressure

Having hypertension or abnormally high blood pressure is a very serious condition.

Your life expectancy is shortened, even by moderately high levels, due to your heightened risk for … stroke (haemorrhage or blood clot in the brain) … heart attack (interruption of the blood supply to a part of the heart which causes heart cells to die) … heart failure (reduced pumping ability) … atherosclerosis (narrowing of the arteries) … aneurysm (in which a balloon-like bulge in an artery can rupture) … kidney disease (in which the kidneys fail to adequately filter waste products and toxins from your blood so that you end up with internal poisoning), and …eye damage.

Extremely high blood pressure can be deadly. All the medical websites I visited warn that if your blood pressure is 50% or more above the average, you can expect to live no more than a few years unless you have it treated.

It doesn't take much nous to figure out that controlling your blood pressure is vital, and that you have to take steps to ensure that your readings are 115/75mmHg or less.

If you have hypertension you can be sure that you are not unique. Statistics suggest that at least 20% of the people in the Western world have been diagnosed as having hypertension.

However, as the condition does not show any symptoms until complications have occurred, it is likely that many more people have hypertension but are not aware of it. Some researchers believe that the number of people with hypertension in the developed world is about 40%.

How do you control you blood pressure?

Firstly you have to monitor it, and then take the appropriate medical measures if it is too high.

Monitoring your blood pressure

You can have you blood pressure monitored by your healthcare provider or you can take and record readings yourself at home.

Having your blood pressure taken by a professional usually entails a visit to a clinic or doctor's office which can be time consuming and expensive, and therefore infrequent. According to the American Heart Association, anyone with hypertension should monitor his or her blood pressure at home.

In my view, if you have diabetes, controlling your blood pressure is just as important as controlling your glucose and cholesterol levels. Monitoring at home provides you with the information you need and improves the management of your blood pressure levels.

It has several distinct benefits. You can track your treatment to see whether it is effective. It helps to keep you motivated to control your blood pressure through exercise, diet and the proper use of your medicines. It also eliminates white-coat hypertension or anxiety due to visiting a clinic which tends to raise blood pressure.

The only drawbacks I can find with monitoring your blood pressures at home on your own is that you could become obsessed by it and check your blood pressure too often.

Automatic self-contained blood pressure monitors you can use at home are available at reasonable prices. These are usually quite reliable ... provided they are approved for home use and have been independently tested.

Lists of validated monitors are available from the British Hypertension Society (http://bhsoc.org/default.stm) and Dabl Educational Trust (www.dableducational.org) in the USA.

Using a home monitoring device

If you have your blood pressure under good control, you only need to check it on a few days in each month. However, if you are having problems with your diabetes or have recently changed your medications, you may need to monitor it more often.

It is best to carry out several readings at various times during the days you monitor your blood pressure. This way you can calculate your average blood pressure for the day.

Because your blood pressure varies throughout the day, you should take the measurements at the same time of day in order to make sure that the readings are comparable.

To ensure an accurate reading, you should NOT drink coffee, smoke or engage in strenuous exercise for 30 minutes before taking the reading. And you should also urinate, if you need to, as a full bladder can have a small effect on your blood pressure. [Isn't the internet a fascinating place!?]

Each time you check your blood pressure, do it twice, because the first reading may be a little high due to the effort involved in putting on the cuff and setting up the machine.

Always place the cuff around your bare skin, as readings taken over a shirt sleeve are less accurate.

It is important to make sure that both your arm and the measuring cuff are in their correct positions. The arm being used should be relaxed and kept at heart level, for example by resting it on a table.

To make sure your readings are comparable over time, you should always use the same arm (either left or right) when you are measuring your blood pressure. This is because there can be slight differences in blood pressure between the two arms.

However, every now and then, you should measure your blood pressure twice, once in each arm, to check if there is a great difference in the readings between the two arms.

If there is a significant difference in the pressure in one arm compared to the other, this could be due to a narrowing of an artery. This narrowing could be due to one of several serious causes. But don't panic ... the difference may not be due to a narrowed artery. Just contact your clinic soonest.

To be able to see how your blood pressure is faring over time, you need to record the readings, with a manual method or a computer program such as MS Excel.

As well as recording date, time and BP reading, you could also record a note on the kind of activities you had been undertaking in the hour before you took the reading. These notes could prove useful when evaluating the variations in your blood pressure.

Controlling blood pressure
Anyone can suffer from high blood pressure. However, certain factors can seriously worsen your hypertension and increase the risk that you will suffer complications.

These aggravating factors are ... genetic factors (a tendency for hypertension in your family) ... obesity ... smoking ... diabetes ...

kidney diseases ... too much alcohol ... too much salt in your diet ... lack of exercise ... and certain medicines, such as steroids.

As there are no early signs of high blood pressure, if you have a family history of hypertension, you should have regular blood pressure tests as a matter of course, so that any treatment needed can be started before any complications arise.

To bring your hypertension under control, you have two main courses of action: (a) taking prescribed medicines on a regular basis and (b) changing your lifestyle. Both courses of action are vital for your health and longevity.

Prescribed medicines ... if your blood pressure requires medical treatment, you will probably have to take medicine on a regular basis. Medicines for hypertension should only be taken when prescribed by a medical doctor.

Note that if you are on medication for high blood pressure, you should never stop taking it without consulting your doctor, even if you feel fine. Hypertension can lead to very serious complications if it is not treated properly.

Lifestyle changes ... are changes you need to make in order to beat your hypertension. They include ... stopping smoking ... losing weight ... exercising regularly ... eating a low-fat diet ... reducing your consumption of alcohol (even if you are a moderate drinker) ... reducing levels of stress (either by avoiding stressful situations or using relaxation techniques).

These kinds of lifestyle changes need to be taken seriously. Indeed, to reduce your blood pressure, they are absolutely necessary. And, if you are not yet hypertensive, they will reduce your risk of developing high blood pressure.

Without treatment for your high blood pressure, you run a very high risk of developing diseases such as heart failure or stroke and thus reduce your life expectancy and quality of life significantly.

6 - Cholesterol, Triglycerides & Trans-fats

For years I had high levels of cholesterol in my blood ... clogging up my arteries. I didn't know it, as there were no symptoms.

I ended up with *peripheral vascular disease*, a general term for any disorder of the circulatory system outside the area of the heart and brain. High cholesterol, along with neuropathy due to my diabetes, has deadened my feet. There is no cure.

My cholesterol levels are now under control, using prescription drugs and a plant-focused diet. My feet have stopped getting worse. Though there are no cures for peripheral vascular disease and neuropathy, I do seem to be holding my own ... so far.

Most people who have high levels of glucose in their blood also have high levels of cholesterol or triglycerides. To beat your diabetes, you must also tackle your cholesterol and triglycerides.

Cholesterol and triglycerides are both fats, but different kinds of fats. Cholesterol is used to build cells, while triglycerides are used to store energy in the form of unused calories.

Cholesterol

Cholesterol is a microscopic ingredient found in the membranes of animal cells, including humans. Plants do not contain any cholesterol.

Cholesterol is vital for animal life. It holds the thin membranes (sheet-like coverings) of your body cells together ... without cholesterol your body would collapse into a heap like a jelly. It also has a role in sending signals to your cells along your nerves. In addition, it is the raw material your body uses to make certain hormones, as well as vitamin D which controls the calcium in your body.

About 75 to 80% of your cholesterol is made by synthesising other substances inside your own body. Around 25% of this internal production takes place in your liver. Cholesterol is also made in your intestines, adrenal glands and reproductive organs.

The rest comes from the animal products you eat. If you eat too much cholesterol, you body will compensate by reducing the amount of cholesterol it makes ... provided all your systems are working properly. If not, you will end up with too much cholesterol.

Cholesterol is transported from your liver through the blood stream to where it is needed to build cells. Because it is insoluble, it has to be carried within lipoproteins, which are soluble in blood.

Lipoproteins

Lipoproteins are combinations of fats and proteins.

Low-density lipoproteins transport cholesterol from the liver to wherever it has to go. LDL is known as 'bad' cholesterol, because as it trucks along it deposits cholesterol in the linings of your arteries, making it more likely you will develop cardiovascular problems.

High-density lipoproteins mop up excess cholesterol and take it back to your liver for reprocessing. HDL is called 'good' cholesterol because when the levels you have in your blood are raised, you have better protection against heart disease.

Triglycerides

Lipoproteins also transport *triglycerides*, molecules of fat that are used to store unused calories and provide your body with energy. Having triglycerides in your bloodstream is quite normal.

When you eat, your body converts any calories it doesn't need immediately into triglycerides, which are stored in your fat cells. Hormones then release the triglycerides for energy between meals. If you often eat more calories than you use up, it likely you will have high levels of triglycerides.

Cholesterol damage

The level of cholesterol in your body will depend on the amount you are eating and the amount being produced internally by your body. Having a high level of cholesterol in your bloodstream can kill you. Here's why.

When too many particles of cholesterol are being delivered through your arteries by low-density lipoproteins (LDL), they tend to collide and become damaged. These damaged particles cause *plaques* (raised bumps or small scars) to form on the walls of your arteries.

These plaques are fragile. When a plaque ruptures, the blood around it starts to clot. To contain the rupture, the clot will grow. If the clot grows big enough, it will block the artery.

If an artery that carries blood to your heart is blocked, you'll have a heart attack. If the blood vessels in your feet get blocked, you'll end up with deadened feet, which was my fate.

Once you have too much cholesterol in your blood you are on your way to angina, heart disease and stroke. Excess cholesterol can also damage the tiny blood vessels in your eyes and kidneys.

The solution to this threat is to reduce the cholesterol circulating in your bloodstream ... by using prescription drugs that suppress your internal production of cholesterol and by switching to a diet that reduces your intake of cholesterol, which is what I am doing.

Damage from high triglycerides

Too much triglyceride in your blood may cause hardening of the arteries (*atherosclerosis*), making you ripe for a stroke or heart attack, even where cholesterol levels have not been too high. Excessive levels of triglycerides can also lead to inflammation of the pancreas.

High levels of triglycerides in your blood can be due to your genes, obesity, drinking too much alcohol, having diabetes and insulin resistance, certain medications, and a high carbohydrate diet.

There's nothing you can do about your genes. However, you can reduce you weight and the amount you drink, and get your diabetes under control.

A meal in which carbohydrates account for more than 60% of the total calories can increase triglyceride levels temporarily. This effect is stronger for those who are badly over-weight. Thus, if you slim down and eat food that has a low glycemic index (ie, food that releases glucose into the bloodstream slowly) you should have no triglyceride problems with a high carbohydrate diet.

The problem with high cholesterol and triglyceride levels is that you don't get any symptoms ... until damage starts showing up in your heart, arteries, kidneys, eyes and feet.

Meanwhile, diabetes will be reinforcing the damage to your cardiovascular system, kidneys, eyes, and feet and hands.

Measuring cholesterol and fat levels in your blood

As mentioned previously, the amount of glucose, cholesterol and other substances in your blood is measured in the USA in milligrams per decilitre (mg/dl) and in millimoles per litre (mmol/l) in most other places.

The factors for converting mmol/l to mg/dl are as follows:

(a) Cholesterol ... multiply by 38.7
(b) Triglycerides ... multiply by 88.6

Guideline levels
According to both the National Cholesterol Education Program
(NCEP) in the USA and the American Heart Association (AHA),
your level of cholesterol should be less than 5.2mmol/l (200mg/dl) ...
and once it is over 6.2mmol/l (240mg/dl) you should be treated with
cholesterol-lowering drugs.

I discovered that many researchers consider these
recommendations to be too high. The average cholesterol level in the
USA is about 5.3mmol/l (205mg/dl), while heart attacks are causing
about 50% of deaths. A near average level does not look like a good
bet!

Many medical scientists say that HDL and LDL cholesterol
should be tested for separately.

LDL cholesterol ... for diabetics, the recommended level of the
plaque-making cholesterol at which treatment with cholesterol-
lowering drugs should begin is 2.6mmol/l (100mg/dl) in the USA or
2mmol/l (77mg/dl) in the UK.

I was not able to find out why the recommended upper limit is
30% higher in the USA compared to the UK.

But what I did find out is many medical researchers say that the
upper limit for diabetics should be 1.8mmol/l (70mg/dl), and that the
risk of heart problems is minimised when the LDL level is about
1.0mmol/l (40mg/dl).

HDL cholesterol ... as HDL carries cholesterol out of your body, the
higher your HDL level, the better. Actual levels range from
0.5mmol/l (19mg/dl) to 1.6mmol/l (62mg/dl).

Recommended levels are above 1.2mmol/l (45mg/dl) for men and
above 1.4mmol/l (55mg/dl) for women.

Cholesterol ratio ... it's not just the absolute levels of LDL and HDL
cholesterol that count, however. Many researchers are of the opinion
that your HDL as a proportion of your total cholesterol level should
be at least 1/3 of your total cholesterol level, and that the higher it is
the better.

For example, if your total cholesterol level is 3.9mmol/l

(150mg/dl), your HDL level should be at least 1.3mmol/l (50mg/dl), preferably a bit higher.

The cholesterol ratio is important, in my view, because I have found research that indicates that the lower the proportion of HDL in your total cholesterol, the greater your risk of cardiovascular disease. Thus, increasing HDL as a proportion of total cholesterol while reducing overall cholesterol seems to be a better approach compared to just trying to reduce total cholesterol.

Triglycerides ... guideline levels from the American Heart Association for concentrations of triglycerides in the blood and associated degrees of risk for medical complications are as follows:

- Low risk ... less than 1.69mmol/l (150mg/dl)
- Medium risk ... 1.70 mmol to 2.25 mmol (150mg/dl to 199mg/dl)
- High risk ... 2.26mmol to 5.65mmol (200mg/dl to 499mg/dl)
- Very high risk ... more than 5.65mmol (500mg/dl)

Thus to feel safe you need to keep your triglycerides below 1.69mmol/l (150mg/dl).

Reducing cholesterol and triglyceride levels
To reduce your levels of cholesterol and triglycerides, changes in your lifestyle are essential. But, as well as changing the way you eat, work, live and play, you may need medication.

Lifestyle changes
You are very likely to have excessive levels of cholesterol and triglycerides if you are diabetic, have high blood pressure, smoke, drink too much alcohol, are obese, don't get much exercise, or eat a lot of saturated fats. You can control all of these factors.

You can beat your diabetes and get your blood pressure under control with the diet that worked for me. As smoking increases your levels of LDL ('bad') cholesterol, giving up smoking is vital. As is reducing your intake of alcohol ... because alcohol is high in sugar and calories, small amounts of alcohol can raise your blood glucose levels and your triglycerides.

Reducing your weight and taking regular exercise is absolutely necessary to lower your cholesterol and triglycerides levels.

Research shows that regular exercise boosts your HDL ('good') cholesterol and reduces both LDL cholesterol and triglycerides.

Dropping just five to ten pounds (two to four kilograms) off your weight will lower your triglycerides significantly.

To complement the lifestyle changes you make, medications may be needed.

Medications for cholesterol and triglycerides

Because 75 to 80% of your cholesterol is created inside your body, the effect of a low-cholesterol diet in reducing your cholesterol level is limited. In addition, your own system will compensate for a reduction in your dietary intake of cholesterol by upping your internal production.

Several prescription drugs are available for the treatment of high cholesterol and these also affect triglyceride levels. They help decrease your LDL ('bad') cholesterol, increase your HDL cholesterol, and decrease your triglycerides. The effects of the various drugs on these three factors vary. Here's what I found out about the most common of these drugs.

Statins ... are most effective in lowering LDL cholesterol. They are only moderately successful in raising HDL and in lowering triglycerides. But statins have also been shown to have a beneficial effect on the arteries ... they help to re-absorb some of the particles deposited in the arteries.

Selective cholesterol absorption inhibitors ... are good at lowering LDL but only moderately successful in raising HDL ('good') cholesterol and in lowering triglycerides, and need to be taken with statins.

Resins ... decrease LDL ('bad') cholesterol.

Fibrates ... are very good for lowering triglycerides.

Omerga-3 fatty acid supplements ... can be effective in lowering cholesterol and triglycerides.

Niacin (nicotinic acid) ... can lower triglycerides and LDL ('bad') cholesterol, and raise HDL cholesterol. However it can cause toxicity, and tends to raise blood glucose levels.

What ever medication you are on, you should only take it in accordance with the instructions of your doctor who will combine various medications for the most effective prescription for your needs. If you have any unexpected side-effects, you should report them immediately to your doctor.

Damage from trans-fats

Trans-fats are vegetable oils that have been processed to create a solid, spreadable fat with an increased shelf life. They cost much less to produce than animal fats. However, trans-fats increase LDL ('bad') cholesterol and lower HDL cholesterol, thus adversely affecting your cholesterol ratio.

Why trans-fats do this is not fully understood. But it seems your body finds it difficult to metabolize trans-fats, so they remain in your blood stream for longer and are therefore more prone to making the deposits in your arteries that form plaques. There is no safe level for their consumption.

In the USA it is estimated that more than 30,000 deaths a year related to coronary disease are due to the consumption of trans-fats. There is evidence that long-term ingestion of trans-fats may cause insulin resistance by interrupting the binding of insulin to the receptors in muscle cells, ie increasing the risk of getting type 2 diabetes.

Trans-fats also enhance the accumulation of fat in the abdomen, which means that they increase your risk of obesity.

Most governments are taking steps to reduce trans-fats in the diets of their populations. They have been banned from restaurants and fast-food shops in some places, in cities such as Calgary and New York.

When Denmark introduced strict regulations governing the use of trans-fats its deaths from ischemic heart disease, in which the flow of blood is reduced, fell by 50%.

Being a manufactured fat, trans-fats can only appear in processed foods ... with modern food-labelling I find it easy to keep trans-fats out of my diet.

7 - Smoking

Smoking is for schmucks ... I was one ... doing two packs a day for nearly 40 years. I now have to live with peripheral vascular disease and a restricted ability to walk.

Like most guys of my generation, it began in school. In those days, smoking was cool, even though the threat of lung cancer from smoking was already well known and had received a lot of publicity.

But we ignored that threat ... being cool was more important.

Once I got to college, I began smoking in earnest. In the billiard-room it was a case of smoke or choke and smoking was expected behaviour. At the end of my first year in college I was doing 20 (one whole pack) a day of Carroll's No 1, Ireland's favourite brand, while discussing the dangers of smoking.

Then the ads for 'Silkcut' came out. Silkcut cigarettes became very popular because (the ads said) they contained 'reduced tar', the cancer-causing ingredient in cigarettes, and therefore were less dangerous. And we believed this crap. Many of us switched to Silkcut.

What the Silkcut ads did not explain is the reduced nicotine in each Silkcut cigarette meant that my craving wasn't satisfied by just one fag and my consumption went up. It didn't take long before I was on 40 a day, getting the same amount of nicotine and tar as before.

After a few months I switched back to my favourite brand in an effort to reduce the drain on my wallet. But the Silkcut-ingrained habit remained and my numbers crept up again ... slowly but surely to 40 a day ... that's two or three an hour. And that's where it remained for the next few decades.

How smoking works

A cigarette contains more than 4000 chemical compounds and at least 400 toxic substances. It burns at about 700 degrees Centigrade at the tip and at 60 degrees C towards the butt.

The active substance in tobacco is nicotine which was once widely used as an insecticide. That's right ... when you light up, you are smoking a bug killer, a toxin that kills creepy-crawlies!

Nicotine causes dopamine, a neurotransmitter associated with pleasure, to be released. This affects the levels of, and balance between, certain chemicals in your brain. These are the chemicals that boost your level of concentration, energy and memory, and alter your mood. This is why smoking is enjoyable.

But there's a catch. Some of the compounds in tobacco cause fundamental changes to your brain chemistry ... and you become dependent on smoking, ie you become a tobacco addict.

Now, here's the second catch. As you smoke, your brain continues to change ... its capacity for nicotine expands continuously under its influence, so you need more and more nicotine to get the same effect. It's not surprising that your consumption goes up.

Once your brain has become dependent on the chemicals in tobacco, it will send out a signal when it wants you to smoke again. If you don't smoke, your brain will deliver a strong urge to smoke. If you refuse to give in, it will make you tense and irritable, that is, you will get withdrawal symptoms. This is why giving up smoking is so extremely difficult.

The good news is that, if you refuse to give in, your brain will readjust itself ... it will give up its need for nicotine ... your withdrawal symptoms will dissipate.

After a time, a day or so, a week or so, of a year or two, depending on your internal make-up, your symptoms will disappear altogether

But they'll be ready to appear again (just as strong as before) should you try even one cigarette.

Damage

The four most damaging substances in cigarettes are:

(a) nicotine, which increases your cholesterol levels and constricts your arteries,
(b) tar, a carcinogen,
(c) carbon monoxide, which reduces your oxygen intake, and
(d) particles of smoke, which clog and destroy your lungs.

Cholesterol issues

Nicotine causes your body to release its stores of fat and cholesterol into your bloodstream. This increases you LDL ('bad') cholesterol and decreases your HDL ('good') cholesterol. It also increases your triglycerides slightly.

Great ... if what you want is clogged arteries!

Cancers

The tar in cigarettes contains at least four carcinogens that cause cancer of the lungs, mouth, throat, and bladder, and are contributory causes to cancers of the kidneys, pancreas and cervix.

According to my research, ninety percent of all lung cancer cases are due to smoking. The statistics I found suggest that if you smoke more than 15 cigarettes a day, your chances of dying of lung cancer are at least 1 in 5 (20% +). If you smoke less than 15 a day, your chances are 1 in 10 (still lousy odds). But if you have never touched a cigarette, your changes of getting lung cancer are only 0.5%, ie less than half of one percent.

If you manage to quit permanently, it will take about 15 years before your risk of lung cancer drops to the same level of risk as a non-smoker.

In addition, as a smoker, your risk of getting mouth cancer is four times higher than for a non-smoker.

Cardiovascular diseases

Cardiovascular diseases are the main causes of deaths due to smoking ... nicotine acts as a stimulant, it raises blood pressure, and it is also a vasoconstrictor.

Nicotine stimulates your heart to beat faster and, by raising your blood pressure and constricting your arteries, makes it harder for your heart to deliver the correct amount and speed of blood for whatever you are doing. By raising your blood pressure, smoking can cause hypertension.

Nicotine contributes to atherosclerosis (hardening of the arteries), which makes the formation of blood clots likely. Indeed, if you smoke you are four times more likely to develop blood clots in your heart and brain ... the most common causes of sudden death.

Smoking causes about 30% of coronary thromboses, clots in the arteries leading to the heart which can precipitate heart attacks. The weed is also a prime cause of cerebral thrombosis (blocking of the blood vessels to the brain) which causes strokes and paralysis.

Smoking restricts the blood supply to your kidneys, so your kidneys may fail to control your blood pressure. As the damage worsens you will probably require dialysis and eventually a transplant.

Nicotine also restricts the blood supply to your skin and to your legs and feet, and you end up not being able to walk without resting every few minutes. The outlook, unless you quit smoking and reduce the blockages through diet and exercise, is grim ... gangrene and eventually amputation.

These cardiovascular diseases are also caused by high blood pressure, high levels of cholesterol and triglycerides, and diabetes. Put all these conditions together with smoking (one of the causes of high blood pressure and excess cholesterol levels) and you have a sure-fire recipe for a long drawn-out painful death.

COPD

Chronic obstructive pulmonary disease (COPD) refers to long-term medical conditions that block airflow to the lungs. These include *emphysema*, in which the air sacs in the lungs are damaged, and *chronic bronchitis* or continuous coughing with a lot of mucus.

Smoking is responsible for 80% of all cases of COPD, which affects 94% of all those who smoke one pack of 20 cigarettes a day. Lung damage from COPD is permanent. But, if you give up smoking at any time, you will reduce the rate of decline in your lung capacity.

I watched my father die from emphysema. It began as breathlessness that slowly got worse over ten years. Despite a pump for getting oxygen into his lungs, his body eventually wasted away. At the end he was so light, I could almost lift him with one hand. He died painfully from lack of air.

After seeing him die, I continued to smoke for another twenty years.

Other damage

Smoking dramatically increases the risk of other serious medical conditions ... impotence ... cataracts (which makes the eyes cloudy) ... and macular degeneration (with a gradual loss of eyesight).

If you have asthma, smoking will make it worse and counteract any medicines you are taking to ease the condition. It also increases the risk of dental diseases, such as bad breath, swollen gums and falling teeth, and contributes to the development of mouth ulcers.

You don't need a degree in rocket science to work it out ... if you smoke, you must quit ... permanently.

Giving up

There are two things you need to tackle if you are to quit smoking permanently … your physical addiction (which will cause real physical symptoms when you stop giving your body nicotine) … and your psychological dependency (which can only be broken by changing your habits).

Researching the internet, I found lots of advice (some of it sage, some less wise) on how to quit smoking. You can (i) give up gradually, (ii) go cold turkey, (iii) use nicotine replacement therapy, (iv) use drugs, or (v) try alternative treatments such as acupuncture and hypnosis.

Giving up gradually

I tried giving up smoking by cutting down progressively. It didn't work for me.

But I do know that it does work for some people. What they do is avoid smoking in situations where they habitually smoke, such as having a cup of coffee, after a meal, watching TV and so on.

When they do this, the nicotine-craving signals from their brain reduce gradually.

Try it. You'll probably find that all the will-power you need would be better employed quitting once and for all, suddenly and finally.

Going cold turkey

Quitting suddenly … once and for all … is probably the most effective way to give up smoking permanently.

But it is hell. I've been there ... it takes more willpower than I could muster. But I do know people who quit by going cold turkey. They suffered the horrors.

Quitting suddenly is easy for the first twenty minutes or so. But as the usual time for your next cigarette passes, you experience a gale of cravings. It takes guts to ignore these cravings. It also takes a lot of understanding from your friends and family as you become ultra-irritable.

According to my research, the consensus of opinion is that your physical withdrawal symptoms will peak after about 24 hours and then gradually ease over the following 2 to 4 weeks. I'm not sure whether this is true. When I tried to go cold turkey, I was still freaking out several days after I quit.

Your cravings, however, will eventually die down and cease entirely. Then you are free ... provided you never touch another cigarette in your whole life.

If you do smoke just once, you'll be back where you started. It only takes one cigarette for your cravings to be reinstated and to reach the peak they had previously.

Nicotine replacement therapy

Nicotine replacement therapy (NRT) is a way of getting nicotine into your bloodstream without smoking. It replaces the nicotine you would otherwise be getting from cigarettes. You have a wide choice ... gums ... patches ... inhalers ... lozenges ... and sprays.

Nicotine gum is popular but the risk of becoming dependent on the gum is quite strong. It happened to me. Then you need to cut down on the gum, which is not as hard as cutting down on smoking.

Nicotine patches are in vogue, perhaps because they can be worn discretely under the shirt-sleeves. Personally, I found them to be useless. Perhaps my thick skin doesn't absorb nicotine very well.

A nicotine inhaler is a fake cigarette into which you insert a nicotine cartridge. You use it just like a cigarette except you don't have to light-up. I have never used one. But I have been told that they are handy if you miss the hand-to-mouth movements and labial action of real smoking.

Nicotine lozenges are another way for getting nicotine absorbed through the lining of your mouth. You put a lozenge under your tongue and let it dissolve. I have never used them.

Nicotine nasal sprays are another replacement therapy I have not tried. You insert the sprayer in a nostril, spray and inhale to get a dose of nicotine. You absorb the nicotine quickly through the lining of your nose. I understand that this is useful for relieving sudden surges of the craving to smoke.

However, there is a risk you will become dependent on the nicotine-replacement product you use. This happened to me. Maybe I'm just unlucky. But it seems obvious to me that once your body has become addicted to nicotine (no matter how it's delivered) it will continue to crave the drug until you just stop giving in to your brain.

All NRT does is replace one way of getting nicotine into your system with another. It maintains your dependence on the drug. But switching to nicotine replacement therapy does reduce your risk of lung cancer significantly.

Yet it also means that you body is continuing to release its stores of fat and cholesterol into your bloodstream and the damage to your arteries is continuing. You still have the increased risk of hypertension that is the lot of smokers, and a host of other risks.

Drugs

When giving up smoking I did not use any drugs. However through research I did find out that there is one drug that is helpful, the anti-depressant bupropion. The brand name is Zyban.

You can only get Zyban on prescription from a doctor or smoking clinic. It is not an entirely safe drug and, depending on the dose, could make you more likely to have a seizure. However it does double your chances of still being off cigarettes three months after you've given them up.

Alternative treatments

Other ways of giving up smoking include hypnotherapy and acupuncture.

Frankly, I don't see how hypnotherapy could work. How can suggestions, no matter how strong, prevent the occurrence of physical cravings without some form of physical intervention?

And I tried acupuncture years ago. It didn't work either.

Tackling psychological dependency

Overcoming the mental reasons why you smoke may be just as important as killing your physical craving for tobacco. For this you need some form of human support.

You should also try to avoid situations where smoking almost seems natural, when, for example, drinking coffee, reading the newspaper, hanging out with friends. Becoming a monk or a nun might be helpful too.

Fear is a great motivator. What I did was list the reasons why I wanted to give up smoking. The only ones I could think of were to avoid certain diseases. So my list ended up looking something like this:

- avoid lung cancer ... survival rate for 5 years after diagnosis only 5% (lousy odds)
- avoid emphysema ... the death it delivers is a sort of slow, painful

strangulation
- avoid clogged arteries from excessive cholesterol
- avoid damaged kidneys
- avoid heart attacks
- avoid strokes
- slow the development of PVD (peripheral vascular disease)

Making a very specific list like this worked for me ... after a fashion. You should make a similar list.

What I did to give up smoking

After smoking for just over 40 years, I have given up entirely.

I was hospitalised in 2005 in order to have a by-pass operation around an aneurism just above my left knee. The medics discovered that I had peripheral vascular disease caused by smoking.

I tried going cold turkey. It didn't work. Within a short time of leaving the hospital I was back on 40 fags a day ... stupid. So I wrote out my list of reasons and tried cutting down ... it didn't really work either. I'd get my consumption down a bit and then, as I relaxed, it sneaked back up.

Then I discovered Nicorette, an anti-smoking gum. It helped enormously. I was able to give up cigarettes, except for the occasional few. Then, one day, I decided no more cigarettes, just the gum. Giving up cigarettes entirely was not too difficult at this stage. But I was hooked on Nicorette. I was still getting my doses of nicotine.

So I rewrote my list – concentrating on the diseases I was still risking with nicotine. This time the list was a bit shorter (the cancers were off), but it was still formidable. I came off Nicorette gradually. I limited the number of pieces of gum I allowed myself to chew in any one day. I started substituting regular chewing gum. Eventually I succeeded in dropping Nicorette altogether.

It took me more than five years to give up smoking and break my nicotine habit.

Giving up smoking is hard. Most people take four or five attempts before they finally succeed. But it can be done.

The benefits are enormous ... you will reduce your risk of smoking-related illnesses ... your heart will be less strained and more efficient ... you will be able to work and play better ... your general health will improve and you will feel much healthier ... your sense of taste and smell will be heightened dramatically and you'll enjoy food much, much more ... and so on, and on.

Because you have diabetes you, more than likely, also have issues with your blood pressure and the levels of your cholesterol and triglycerides. Giving up smoking and nicotine is a vital part of beating your diabetes.

8 - Exercise Helps

I managed to beat my diabetes and get my blood glucose levels under control without undertaking any exercise programme at all. The diet I am following was enough on its own.

But I have since discovered that exercise can boost the effect of a healthy diet. Exercise, however, cannot make up for a poor diet, and diet is more important than exercise to control diabetes.

But, that said, regular physical exercise is absolutely crucial for controlling your blood pressure, cholesterol and triglycerides. Because you are a diabetic, there is an 85% chance that you have problems in these areas also and exercise will help immensely in getting these under control.

Physical exercise

Physical exercise is any activity that enhances or maintains your physical fitness and overall health and well-being.

There are three broad types of physical exercise: (i) flexibility exercises, (ii) aerobic exercises and (iii) anaerobic exercises.

The differences between them arise on the effect a particular type of exercising has on your body.

(i) Flexibility exercises

Flexibility exercises are stretching exercises. They are designed to maintain the range of motion you have in your joints and muscles, and are used to 'warm-up' before doing any aerobic or anaerobic training. Flexibility exercises can also be used to relieve stress.

Examples include sun-worship and toe-tipping (see below).

(ii) Aerobic exercises

Aerobic exercises are any kind of rhythmic activity performed continuously for a sustained period (at least 10 minutes) at moderate levels of intensity.

Aerobic means 'with oxygen' and the purpose of these exercises is to improve the use of oxygen in your body's energy-generating process.

Examples include walking, hiking, running (but not sprinting), tennis, dancing, skating, swimming, cycling, rope skipping and rowing.

Anaerobic exercises

Anaerobic or resistance exercises are exercises in which the emphasis is on muscular efforts that strengthen your muscles (strength training).

These exercises use resistance to your muscular contractions to build the strength, size and endurance of your muscles.

Examples include push-ups, deep knee bends, training by lifting weights, and sprinting.

Anaerobic and aerobic exercises differ in how energy is generated within your muscles ... due to the differences in the intensity and duration of the muscular contractions involved in the two types of exercises.

Benefits of regular exercise

Researchers have found that frequent and regular aerobic exercise can prevent or treat chronic conditions such as type 2 diabetes, elevated cholesterol levels, high blood pressure, heart diseases, insomnia and mild depression.

Regular exercise can also help you control your weight, keep your muscles strong and your joints supple, and slow down the deterioration in brain function you encounter as you grow older.

The WHO's *Global Recommendations on Physical Activity* outlines how much physical activity people need. For adults this is at least 150 minutes (2.5 hours) of moderately intensive aerobic physical activity a week. Those over 65 need additional activities to enhance their balance on three or more days a week.

Diabetes and exercise

My personal experience has convinced me that exercise can cause blood glucose levels to drop. I have also found that doing a particular exercise before a meal seems to lower blood glucose more than the same exercise after a meal.

I also discovered that, although diet is more effective than exercise in reducing glucose levels after meals, exercise has been shown to reduce HbA1c levels. Thus, the best way to get your blood sugar under control is to combine some form of regular exercise with the plant-focused diet I am eating.

Cholesterol, triglycerides and exercise

Regular exercise will improve your cholesterol profile and reduce your triglyceride levels.

Exercise does not lower total cholesterol, as it has no effect on LDL ('bad') cholesterol. But it will increase your HDL cholesterol (by up to 10%) which improves your overall cholesterol profile.

Moderate physical activity, such as walking, lowers triglyceride concentrations by an average of 0.11mmol/l (10mg/dl). As the normal level for triglycerides in healthy people is less than 1.69mmol/l (< 150mg/dl), this is a significant drop (more than 6.5%).

Strenuous exercising has a greater effect.

Heart disease and exercise

Both aerobic and anaerobic exercises increase the mechanical efficiency of the heart. Aerobic exercise increases cardiac output (the volume of blood being pumped by the heart) and anaerobic strength training increases the thickness of your heart muscles.

The beneficial effects of exercise on the cardiovascular system have been well documented. A study that tracked physical activity among adults with type 2 diabetes over 19 years found that those who undertook at least four hours a week of moderate exercise were about 40% less likely to succumb to heart disease than sedentary people. They also cut their risk of getting a stroke.

Weight control

When you exercise you use energy. So when you start exercising regularly you can expect to lose weight.

This will only happen, or course, if you consume fewer calories than you use up while exercising.

Brain function and exercise

Research has shown that physical activity ... aerobic exercise in particular ... enhances the functioning of the brain in older adults and reduces the risk of developing dementia.

But researchers do not really know why exercise has this effect.

Insomnia and exercise

My research and personal experience show that exercise is a great cure for insomnia ... presumably it's because your muscles demand sleep once they've had a good work-out.

Excessive exercise

During exercising, proteins within muscles are consumed for energy. Fats and carbohydrates are also consumed. Provided you have adequate nutrition and sufficient rest between sessions, your body will renew its tissues at a higher rate than before you began exercising.

Too much exercise, however, can be harmful. Without proper rest, your chances of a stroke or other problem connected with your circulation increases, and your muscle tissue may be slow to develop. This susceptibility to harm will vary between individuals but it will diminish as they get fitter.

My firm advice is that you discuss the matter with your doctor.

Nutrition

The great thing about getting fit is that exercising and eating are mutually exclusive activities. You simple cannot exercise and eat at the same time ... unlike munching in front of the TV.

Proper nutrition is important when you are exercising. A good diet in this context is a one that helps your body to recover after exercise.

Such a diet needs to be well balanced, ie your body must be getting the correct ratio of macro-nutrients (proteins, carbohydrates and fats) whilst also getting plenty of micronutrients (vitamins and minerals).

Some sports nutritionists recommend that you drink an 'engineered recovery beverage' within 30 minutes of finishing an exercise session. I don't know if these drinks are any use. I do know they tend to be rather expensive, certainly much more costly than the plain glass of water I go for.

Flexibility exercising

Getting into regular exercise is thoroughly enjoyable once you have developed the habit. Personally, I follow a rather simple exercise regimen. It seems to work for me, so it should be OK for you too.

I begin with an early morning 'limber-up' (see below). I do this nearly every day when I get up. It consists of three simple flexibility exercises that take less than five minutes in all.

First I do a 'sun-worship' movement ... a yoga movement designed to increase my overall suppleness and flexibility.

I follow this with a knee-bending exercise which I use to the get the circulation moving in my legs so that my blood flows better to my feet. I feel it helps mitigate the effects of the clogged arterioles (a result of smoking and diabetes) which have reduced the sensation in my feet.

Lastly I do a bit of toe-walking, a type of stretching exercise. I'm not sure what this does but it makes me feel good. It rounds off my early morning limber-up flexibility exercises. If you have any problems with your balance, you need to be very careful when trying toe-walking or avoid it altogether.

I also do some stretching exercises before undertaking any aerobic exercises. These consist of two simple actions. In the first, I lean against a wall, my hands flat on the wall and my feet stretched out backwards, so that my body makes an angle of approximately 45 degrees with the wall. I stretch my calf muscles by straightening my knees and bending my ankles.

In the second, I simply stand upright and raise one leg up behind me, bending at the knee. I grab my ankle and bring my foot up as close as it will go to my backside. I repeat with the other leg.

Aerobic exercising

As I had been a wholly sedentary creature for several decades, I began aerobic exercising with just a few brief walks. Eventually I built my walking up to four or five brisk, half-hour walks a week.

Sometimes, when I am short of time, I break my daily half-hour walks up into two or three walks of ten minutes or so each. This seems to be effective in spreading the walking out over the day.

One thing I have discovered is that I cannot skip walking for more than two days in a row. If I do, my fitness seems to dissipate fairly quickly. The difference is noticeable.

Since I took up regular walking, my blood glucose level has been under better control and my energy levels have increased substantially.

You can build walking into your day in several ways. Walk instead of using your car for short trips. Use the stairs instead of lifts.

I now supplement walking with the regular us of an elliptical trainer (or cross-trainer), a stationary exercise machine on which you cycle standing up and holding on to handle bars that move back and forth in synch with your legs.

The great thing about the elliptical trainer is that there no impact on your feet, which you get when your are jogging or running, or indeed walking briskly. You can vary the resistance of the paddle-like pedals from light to very strong. And the machine does not take up too much room.

I use my elliptical trainer on an on-off basis throughout the day … for a few minutes at a time to give me a break from my desk. It adds up to 10 minutes a day, to which I add one 20–30 minute walk.

Resistance exercising

The American Diabetes Association (ADA) recommends that type 2 diabetics (who are otherwise healthy) do resistance exercising … three days a week … covering all major muscle groups.

Resistance exercising involves doing push-ups or similar exercises, lifting weights or using exercise equipment that you push against, squeeze, stretch or bend. In these exercises you progressively overload your musculoskeletal system to make it stronger, ie you go as far as you can on a particular exercise and then back off.

For weight-lifting, the ADA recommends that your work-outs should include three sets of 8 to 10 repetitions at a weight that cannot be lifted more than 8 to 10 times … three times a week.

You don't have to attend a gym. There are plenty of exercises you can do without equipment, such as push-ups or sit-ups. You can also keep a set of weights at home (like we do) as these are easy to tidy away and are one the best ways of developing strength in your upper body.

Early morning limber up

These three get-yourself-going-in-the-morning exercises take no more than 6 minutes.

Sun-worship … stand upright, legs slightly apart and hands hanging loosely down by your side. While breathing in, move your hands slowly out from the sides of your body, raising them gently until they are stretched straight up over your head and almost touching.

Pause. Then, while releasing your breath, bring your hands down slowly in front of your body until they are fully extended pointing down to your toes. Bend your body forward until your finger tips are as near to your toes as possible and let your head hang loosely down from your neck.

Pause until you need to breathe in. Then reverse the movement, ie, breathing in slowly, raise your hands up until they are again stretched straight up over your head.

Pause. Then, exhaling slowly, bring you hands back out and down to your sides again (the position in which you began).

Repeat the entire movement three times.

Note ... ideally you should be able to touch your toes when you are bent over with your hands hanging down in front of your body, but most people cannot do this (me included).

Knee-bending ... stand with your legs a bit apart and your hands down by your side. Go down on your hunkers, slowly, bending your knees as far as they will go. Then rise up again.

As you go down, your hands should be hanging straight down. You can rest your hands on your legs just above the knees to keep your balance if you wish. Eventually you will be able to do the movement with your arms hanging down and keep going until the palms are flat on the floor.

Repeat several times. Build up your ability until you are able to do 10 repetitions.

Note ... the degree to which you can go down on your hunkers will increase over time. Don't force it. Eventually you will be able to hunker down until the palms of your hands are flat on the floor.

Toe-walking ... raise your hands straight up over your head and look at the ceiling. Breathe in and raise yourself up onto your toes, bending your feet at the toe joint. Walk across the room on your raised feet, your eyes on the ceiling, turn, and come back several times, breathing in and out slowly and calmly.

Stop when you have crossed the room several times or have toe-walked for more than 30 metres.

Warning ... check the floor for obstructions before you start, as ideally you should be looking at the ceiling throughout.

9 - Weight Control

When I was growing up we ate mainly fresh, unprocessed foods at home so my waistline measured about 27 inches (just under 70cm) when I left school.

But in college I began eating in student cafés and by the time I was in my early twenties, my waistline was nearing 34 inches (86cm). Despite the fast-food diet favoured by young accountants, I maintained this girth until I was nearing my 40s.

Then I became an international consultant ... and my weight started creeping up. It's amazing how much extra food you can eat when you are on a generous expense account!

When I became trapped in Kuwait when Saddam Hussein invaded in August 1990, my waistline was 38 inches (96.5cm) and I weighed 94kg (207lbs), and had a gut that hung out over my trouser-belt.

From the weight-control point of view, the invasion did me (and many like me) a power of good. A dire shortage of food, and a high degree of anxiety as we kept out of sight to avoid becoming one of Saddam's Guestages, was (in retrospect) a very effective weight-reduction programme. In about two months, my weight dropped from an obese 94kg to an underweight 72kg (159lbs). Strangely, it did not do me any harm and I felt kind of good and more energetic at the lower weight.

Then, after the war, as I got back into business, my weight started to creep up again. After another decade or so, my weight was a fairly consistent 85kg (187lb), fluctuating up and down just a bit every now and then.

When I was diagnosed with diabetes I was advised to lose weight. I tried. Every now and then I'd manage to get it down to nearly 80kg or so (about 175lb) but it kept creeping back up again.

When I finally decided it was time to get serious about beating my diabetes and switched to the plant-focused diet that I am describing in this book, my weight was 85kg (187lb). Nothing happened for about three weeks. Then, suddenly, I started losing weight.

My weight just rolled off ... at a rate of about 2kg (5lbs) a week.

The drop-off slowed as my weight reached below 79kg (174lb) and tapered off entirely at 75kg (165lb). It has held fairly steady ever since, and I feel good and energetic.

Even better, my BMI reading (see below) is now in the middle of the normal range and my average blood glucose, cholesterol and blood pressure levels have also stabilised at 'normal' levels.

Measuring obesity

Obesity is a medical condition in which you have so much body fat that it may have an adverse effect on health. But how do you know whether you are obese or not?

Common sense suggests that the 'correct' weight for a healthy individual will vary depending on his or her physique. Thus, merely measuring you weight in kilograms or pounds is not enough. You need to take your physique into account.

This you can do using the body-mass index (BMI), which allows you to judge (somewhat inaccurately) whether your weight is 'correct' for your size and shape.

Body mass index

Your body mass index is calculated by a simple formula ... your body weight (in kilograms) divided by the square of your height (in metres).

For example, if you weigh 80kg and are 1.8m tall, your BMI would be $80/(1.8 \times 1.8) = 24.7$, a simple number.

Your BMI does not actually measure the percentage of body fat you have. It is only a simple number that shows you how fat or thin you are. It is very rough-and-ready ... as it fails to take factors such as the size of your frame and how muscular you are into account.

Nevertheless, the BMI is used by most medical professionals to determine whether the weight of an individual is too low, normal, or too high.

The guidelines of the World Health Organisation (WHO) classify a person's BMI as follows:

- Severely underweight ... < 16
- Underweight ... 16 - 20
- Normal ... 20 - 25
- Overweight ... 25 - 30
- Obese ... 30 - 35

- Severely obese ... 35 - 40
- Morbidly obese ... > 40

These ranges of BMI only apply to ethnic Europeans, Africans, Arabs and South Asians (ie, Pakistanis and Indians). Ethnic populations in the Far East develop health problems at lower BMIs than Caucasians and Africans.

To take into account the smaller skeletal size and muscularity of their Asian populations compared to Caucasians and Negroes, some Far Eastern countries use different cut-off points.

In Japan and Singapore, for example, a BMI of 18.5 to 23 is considered the normal range. Obesity begins at 25 for the Japanese, while Singaporeans are considered obese if they have a BMI of 27.5 or more.

BMI Prime
BMI Prime is the ratio of your actual BMI number to the upper limit of 'normal' BMI, which is 25 if you are an ethnic Caucasian, Negro or Semite. It is a handy way to find out how much you are over or under 'normal' weight.

For example, if your BMI is 28, you can divide 28 by 25 to get 1.12 ... this means you are overweight by 12%. If your BMI is 35, you divide 35 by 25 to get 1.40 ... which means you are 40% overweight.

If your BMI Prime is between 0.75 (20/25) and 1.00 (25/25), your weight is normal. However, if it is less than 0.75 (eg, 16/25 = 0.64) you are under weight and need to start eating more.

If you are Japanese or Singaporean, instead of dividing by 25 you divide by 23 (the upper limit of 'normal' for people with a Far Eastern physique).

Damage
If you are overweight, your body has more fat cells than your physique (shape and size) warrants, and you risk getting a variety of related diseases including ... type 2 diabetes ... cardiovascular diseases ... several types of cancer ... and fatty liver disease.

Increases in your body fat will alter your body's response to insulin, which can lead to insulin resistance, ie diabetes. Researchers have discovered that excess body fat underlies 64% of cases of diabetes in men and 77% of cases in women.

Being overweight will also increase you blood pressure, cholesterol and triglyceride levels, which is why it puts you at risk of cardiovascular diseases. Common sense suggests that weight control is an important factor in tackling heart diseases of all kinds.

Thus, if you are overweight and are serious about beating your diabetes (which means getting your insulin sensitivity, blood pressure, cholesterol and triglycerides under control) you have to get your weight down. Here are some statistics to get you motivated:

- Large-scale studies of Americans and Europeans have found that the risk of dying is lowest among non-smokers whose BMIs range from 20 to 25 (ie, who are not overweight).
- A 16-year study of women has shown that those with BMIs of more than 32 died at twice the rate of women with BMIs of less than 32.
- In the USA, obesity (BMI >30) causes more than 365,000 deaths a year, while in the EU, excess weight (BMI >25) is a contributory factor in one million (7.7%) of all deaths each year.
- If you are obese, your life expectancy is reduced by an average of six to seven years, ie, a BMI of 30 to 35 reduces life expectancy by two to four years, while extremely severe obesity (BMI > 40) reduces it by 10 years.

With these kinda figures, you just gotta get serious about reducing your weight.

Causes of obesity
The causes of obesity are simple ... a combination of eating too many dietary calories with a lack of physical activity.

Two simple causes ... therefore ... a two-pronged simple solution: (a) change your diet to reduce the calories you eat, and (b) take up regular exercising to increase the calories you use up.

But, to be sure your efforts to diet and exercise are bearing fruit, you have to keep track of your weight.

Monitoring your weight
Tracking your weight is easy. All you need is a regular bathroom scales. But note:

Same time ... you should weigh yourself at the same time each day, as eating and drinking will cause your weigh to go up and down a bit during the day. We are usually at our heaviest in the evening, so weigh yourself when you get up in the morning after you have been to the toilet.

Same scales ... you should use the same weighting scales each time you weigh yourself, as most weighting scales vary a bit.

Calibrate ... always calibrate the scale to zero before you weigh yourself, to ensure that you get comparable readings each time. Most domestic bathroom scales have a little wheel on the side for doing this and they are simple to use.

Reducing weight
Changing your diet (both the type and quantity of food you eat) and physical exercise are the main and best ways to reduce your weight.

If you find dieting too difficult, you can use anti-obesity drugs. These are designed to either reduce your appetite or inhibit how your absorb fat. My strongest possible advice would be to steer clear of these drugs until you have discussed them with your doctor and he has prescribed them for you.

As a final option you can try surgery to reduce the volume of your stomach and/or the length of your bowels by cutting out a section of these internal organs or by inserting an intra-gastric balloon. The result, in both cases, is that you feel satiated quicker and your ability to absorb nutrients is reduced. It's definitely a last resort.

Exercising
The relationship between exercising regularly and losing weight is simple.

If you burn more calories than you eat, you will lose weight ... and if you eat more than you burn, you will gain weight.

Using exercise to reduce weight is harder than changing your diet. To burn off 300 to 400 calories, for example, you need to go on a 3 to 4 mile (6.5km) run. For most people this is not possible on a daily basis.

In my view, changing your diet will be more effective than exercising for reducing your weight. This is how I did it myself. But I am still in favour of regular exercising for all the other benefits it brings.

Diet

Reducing your weight through diet is a cinch. Believe me ... you don't have to count calories ... you don't have to control the amount you eat ... no portion control necessary!

All you have to do is switch the kinds of foods you eat ... change from a Western diet full of fat-rich, high-sugar processed foods to a quasi-vegan diet ... and then eat as much as you like. Provided you stick to the quasi-vegan diet, the amount of food you eat will be controlled automatically.

And you'll love the tastes and textures of a quasi-vegan diet.

This works. It's how I did it ... and went from 85kg (187lb) to 75kg (165lb) in just 10 weeks or so.

In fact, putting your intake of food on 'auto-control' by switching to a quasi-vegan plant-focused diet will probably reduce your daily intake by 300 to 400 calories ... just as much as a daily 3 to 4 mile run ... without any real effort on your part.

The diet I advocate (because it worked for me) is effective in reducing your weight because it is strictly low fat. In summary, it means ... reducing animal fats to a bare minimum by drastically reducing the animal products (meat, fish, milk and dairy products) you eat ... eating plant-based foods, but avoiding seeds, olives, avocados, nuts and full-fat soy products because they are all high in fat ... minimising the use of vegetable oils ... reducing consumption of energy-dense foods (see below), such as processed foods which are high in fat and sugars, and ... eating plenty of high-fibre foods (at least 40 grams a day) with an emphasis on beans and vegetables.

This is essentially the diet I use to beat my diabetes.

Losing weight through a change in diet has several benefits for beating your diabetes ... it makes your cells more responsive to insulin (especially when fat is removed from your waistline) ... it reduces your blood pressure ... it brings down your levels of cholesterol and triglycerides ... and it makes exercising easier (which is something I am all for).

A *vegan diet* is one in which all animal products (meat, fish, milk, yoghurt, cheese, butter, etc, even low-fat varieties) are avoided strictly. The diet I use is only *quasi-vegan*. I still eat a bit of fish and some meat, but only the leanest of lean meat from which I cut out any fat I can see.

My internet research indicates that an average person who goes on a vegetarian diet (and sticks to it) will lose about 10% of his or her body weight. In fact, I dropped more than that (about 11.5%) from 85kg to 75kg on the quasi-vegan diet I now use regularly.

That same average person will lose weight, according to research, at a rate of about 1/2 a kilogram (one pound) a week. In fact, I dropped 10 kilograms in about 8 to 10 weeks, double that rate.

The reason why both a strictly vegan diet and my quasi-vegan diet result in dramatic weight loss is probably because the diet has very little fat, the main source of unwanted calories.

In addition, by eating a plant-focused diet you are ingesting plenty of fibre which is filling and turns off your appetite quicker. Each gram of fibre is said to cut an average of about 10% off your intake of calories.

The two diets also increase your after-meal-calorie-burn slightly. The *after-meal-calorie-burn* refers to the fact that the digestive process itself causes you to burn calories at a faster rate after a meal. A low-fat plant-focused diet speeds this up a bit.

Populations in the Far East who eat plant-based diets, ie carbohydrate-rich foods such as rice and noodles, show few signs of obesity and diabetes, even though they ignore the amount of food they eat (they eat as much as they can when they can get it).

It seems that having the correct foods on your plate (ie plant-based foods), and only using animal products as condiments, means that the amounts they eat automatically fall into line with their requirements for calories and they achieve their correct body weights without any fuss or bother over counting calories or whatever.

Besides my quasi-vegan diet or a full-fledged vegan diet, there are several other diets you can try which may help you lose weight (no sarcasm intended).

ADA diet

The diet recommended by the American Diabetes Association relies on calorie limits ... you have to limit the number of calories you eat each day. For example, if your usual diet is 2000 calories a day, you have to reduce your intake to (say) 1500 calories a day.

Easy? It certainly is ... if you are an expert in nutrition and are able to judge how many calories are contained in each of the hundreds of different kinds of food you could eat.

For the rest of us ... it's almost impossible. I haven't a clue as to how many calories I eat and I really don't know how I could find out with any degree of certainty. I'm sure you're in the same boat. The ADA diet is just not designed for non-experts in nutrition.

As well as requiring you to judge the number of calories you are eating, the ADA diet means that, once you reach your calorie limit for the day, that's it. You stop eating. If you are hungry in the evening, you have to go to bed hungry.

With a vegan or quasi-vegan diet your intake is on 'auto-control' so you can eat whenever you feel hungry and never have to go to bed on an empty stomach.

Low-carb diets
In a low carbohydrate diet you restrict the carbohydrates you eat. This means that you eat more protein ... which, when it comes from animal and dairy products, is high in fat and cholesterol.

Low-carb diets, however, have been shown to be effective in weight-loss. But this loss of weight is usually not permanent and weight returns. In addition, researchers have discovered that low-carb diets have unpredictable health effects.

Weight loss normally lowers cholesterol. According to scientists, a loss of one pound causes cholesterol levels to drop 0.3mmol/l (1mg/dl) on average. The exception is low-carbohydrate diets; they are so high in fat and cholesterol that they increase LDL ('bad') cholesterol levels for about one-third of dieters.

Low-carb diets are also high in animal protein, which is hard on the kidneys and can, if too much is eaten, cause a loss in kidney function.

These diets can be disastrous for diabetics as they are based on the idea that avoiding carbohydrates is the key to controlling your glucose. While it is true that reducing your carbohydrate intake may reduce the amount of glucose released into your bloodstream as part of your digestion process, this method does not address the cause of your insensitivity to insulin ... fat blocking the insulin receptors in your muscle cells.

The fact is, if you have type 2 diabetes, you can only control you glucose levels (in 90% of cases) by reducing the fat in your diet and thereby unblocking your cells' insulin receptors.

Balanced-portions
Balancing the portions of food on your plate is not a form of dieting

as such. Rather, it's a way of ensuring the amounts of three main food types you eat ... animal products, carbohydrates, and vegetables and fruit ... are in balance. You can use it with any sort of diet.

Essentially, you mentally divide your dinner plate into three parts, rather like the 'peace' sign, with three lines radiating out from the centre to the rim of the plate. You assign one part to each of the three main types of food.

For a calorie-counting diet (such as recommended by the ADA), you would probably divide the plate up into three equal segments (33% each) so that each of the main food types would constitute about third of your meal. For a low-carb diet, you might reduce the carbohydrate section to 20% and up the animal products section to 40% or 50%, with the balance going to the vegetables and fruit.

Of course, if you pile one section higher than the other, your food will be out of balance.

For a vegan, the animal products section will be zero and the plate will only be divided into two sections. For the quasi-vegan diet I'm using, about 10% should be OK for the animal product segment. You could have up to 25% for carbohydrates and the rest (65%) for plant-based foods (legumes, vegetables and fruit) other than grains.

I'm not sure that this technique is much good but it does help you consider that you are eating. And bear in mind that it cannot be used to balance the portions of the types of food you put in a bowl with liquids, such as soup.

Calories in food (energy-density)
Body fat is a calorie-storage system. This is true for all animals, including humans.

In rural Africa and Asia, people still eat their traditional diets. These diets are based on grains, root vegetables and legumes, which are filling but contain relatively few calories. Those who eat these kinds of diets tend to be slim.

In Europe and North America our usual diets are based on meat and diary products which contain the calories stored in animal fat. No wonder most of us are overweight.

The facts are ... a gram of animal fat (such as chicken fat) or vegetable oil contains 9 calories ... while a gram of carbohydrate (the starch in rice, beans, yams, etc) only has 4 calories.

Thus, for the same weight, carbohydrates contain less than half the calories found in animal fat. Just by switching from animal products to carbohydrates, you can reduce your calorie-intake by more than 50%.

Vegetable oils, like animal fats, contain 9 calories per gram. However, they are lower in saturated fat than animal fats and therefore must be preferred over animal fats for cooking purposes. However, their use needs to be minimised because of their fat content.

Most foods from plants (grains, beans, vegetables and fruits) contain very little fat, so you can eat as much of these as you like and still remain slim. The exceptions are seeds, olives, avocados, nuts and some soy products which do contain a lot of fat ... and so should be avoided.

Fibre content

The quasi-vegan diet I have found so healthy emphasises foods high in fibre (or roughage as it used to be called) ... at least 40 grams a day.

Many foods have their natural fibre content 'processed out'. For example, a natural grain of rice has a thin coating of fibre that gives it its brown colour, and this is turned into white rice by stripping off the coating and, as a result, white rice has very little fibre.

When you are trying to lose weight, high-fibre foods are very useful as they fill you up more and make you feel full quicker than low-fibre foods. Researchers have estimated that for every 14 grams of fibre you add to your diet will cut your calorie-intake by an average of 10%.

Beans, vegetables, fruits and whole grains have the most fibre. However there is more fibre in beans and most other vegetables than in whole grains. If you want to slim down, beans are the way to go.

Statistics show that people who eat beans regularly weigh, on average, 6.5 pounds (3kg) less than non-bean eaters. Teenagers who eat beans regularly weigh 7 pounds (3.2kg) less and have waistlines nearly one inch slimmer than non-bean eating teens, according to the US National Nutrition & Health Examination Survey (1999-2002).

More recently, researchers at the University of Kentucky combined the results of 11 previous studies and confirmed that bean-eaters are thinner on average.

Energy-density & volumetrics

A really good tip for losing weight (and keeping it off) is to eat foods that make you feel full quicker and also contain fewer calories than your usual food.

Satiety is the feeling of fullness you have after a meal. Unless you are a glutton, you will stop eating once you feel satiated.

Researchers at Pennsylvania State University have discovered that it is the weight of the food we eat that brings on satiety ... not the amount of protein or carbohydrate, or the number of calories, we have taken in.

It is as if your stomach had an internal set of weighting-scales which, once it has registered a certain weight of food, signals 'enough'. Thus, to lose weight, you need to eat food that makes you satiated earlier and is low in calories.

The term *energy-density* describes how many calories are packed into a set amount of a particular food. Water does not contain any calories. Therefore, food that has a lot of water in it has a low energy density ... it contains few calories per gram. And water is relatively heavy.

Volumetrics refers to eating foods that bring on the sensation of satiety with reduced calories by eating foods that contain relatively more water than other foods. The volumetric dieting trick is to eat foods that have low energy-density but are also filling ... foods containing lots of water.

Most people eat about the same weight of food each day. If you eat a bit less, your appetite causes you to eat a bit more. By switching from 'drier' foods to 'waterier' foods, you can take in the same weight of food every day but fewer calories (and feel just as full as usual).

Strangely, just drinking a glass of water before you eat will not reduce your appetite. Nobody seems to know why but water on its own does not seem to register on your internal weighting-scales.

However adding water to other foods (such as casseroles) does increase their weight and brings down their energy density and thus the number of calories in a given weight of that food.

So you can lose weight by switching to low energy-density foods. And there are plenty of low energy-density foods about that are also filling, ie make you feel satiated easily. These include:

- broths ... but not cream soups
- vegetables ... such as tomatoes, cucumbers, peppers, chickpeas

- fresh fruits ... such as apples, pears and oranges which are relatively heavy but contain few calories (but not dried fruits which (by definition) do not contain any water)
- beans
- whole grains ... in the form of rice and pasta which are water-based and filling (but not rice cakes and bread).

Airy foods, such as bread, pretzels, Melba toast and rice cakes, are not high in calories but will not bring on satiety ... you have to eat a lot just to get full.

Fatty foods, such as cheese, onion rings, potato crisps and meat are filling but they contain 9 calories per gram, that is, they have a relatively high energy-density.

Shopping ... you can check out the energy-density of commercial food products just by looking at the label. If the food contains less than one calorie per gram, it has a low energy-density ... the weight of the food will fill you up before the calories fill you out.

The label will show you the number of calories per gram. If not, it will show the number of grams per serving and the number of calories per serving, so you can easily work out the number of calories in a gram of the food.

For example, a tin (can) of spinach may contain 115 grams per serving and 30 calories per serving, so it will contain $30/115 = 0.26$ calories per gram, ie a low energy-density as it less than one. Or, a slice of white bread might weigh 32 grams and deliver 80 calories; thus its calories per gram would be 2.5, ie it has a high energy-density.

There is no need to do the mental arithmetic in your head. Just look at the label ... if number of grams per serving is higher than the number of calories per serving then that food has an energy-density that is less than one, ie is low.

You will find that choosing foods that naturally contain a good amount of water will help you to lose weight. Volumetrics is a handy way for picking the most filling foods with the fewest calories ... and shows us that the best way to reduce weight and keep it off is to eat a plant-based diet.

Medications

The medications you take may affect your ability to control your weight. You need to check the side-effects that are usually listed in the leaflets that you find inside the packaging of your medications.

If you feel that your medications are affecting your ability to reduce or maintain your weight, you must discuss the matter with you doctor thoroughly and take his advice.

Warning ... it would be the height of foolishness to reduce your medications without the explicit advice of the qualified healthcare professional whose job is to help you maintain your health.

Section Two: Diet Essentials

Children who grow up getting nutrition from plant foods rather than meats have a tremendous health advantage. They are less likely to develop weight problems, diabetes, high blood pressure and some forms of cancer ... Benjamin Spock

The purpose of this section is to present the information I feel is needed to make informed decisions when choosing what foods to eat.

Warning: all the information in this section was obtained through research on the internet. As such, it may not be wholly accurate. However, this basic information of foods helped me to devise the diet I am using to beat my diabetes.

10 - My Diet

*Eat: ... natural ... low sugar ... low fat ... low salt ... high fibre ...
low GI ... mostly plants ... all you want ... with lots of water*

The vision of my diet is to beat diabetes by avoiding the risks associated with the disease. Its mission is to reduce the excess amounts of glucose floating around in your bloodstream and get your blood pressure, cholesterol and triglycerides under control.

Because the fundamental problem causing diabetes appears to be fat blocking the receptors in muscle cells, leaving sugar and insulin swirling around aimlessly in your blood, you can beat diabetes by eating foods that are (1) low in sugar, (2) low in fat, (3) low in salt, (4) high in fibre and (5) digested slowly. The easiest way to do this is by concentrating on natural, unprocessed foods that are mostly plants. You also need to drink plenty of water.

The great thing about my diet is that you can eat as much as you want ... no calorie counting ... no restrictions on portion size ... no going to bed on an empty stomach at night.

With this diet you never need to feel hungry ... now, ain't that super cool? Above all, this diet is not about how much you eat ... it's all about what you eat.

All you have to do to beat your diabetes is to eat ... as much as you like of:

- natural, unprocessed foods, mainly plants, that are
- low in sugar
- low in fat
- low in salt
- high in fibre
- digested slowly

But EXCLUDING:
- all dairy products
- all eggs

You also need to drink plenty of water, to aid the absorption of the fibre you eat. Personally I drink at least two litres of water a day in addition to the water, juices, tea and soy milk in my food and coffee.

You should also take a range of supplements in order to cover any possible dietary deficiencies you might encounter by avoiding dairy products.

Believe me it works. All you have to do is learn to read food labels and follow the diet accordingly.

Exercise is not necessary at all to control your blood glucose levels, but it does improve results. But exercise is absolutely necessary to control your blood pressure and cholesterol problems.

Remember ... all your tastes, with the exception of mother's milk, are acquired tastes.

11 - Processed Food

In food processing, harvested crops or butchered animals are used as the raw ingredients for making and packaging food products that are attractive, marketable and have long-shelf lives.

Attractive means that the product both tastes and looks good. To be marketable, it must match the kinds of food being demanded by consumers. Food products that have a long-shelf life reduce the costs of wastage for producers, distributors and retailers.

Despite rumours to the contrary and the shrill shrieks of food faddists, processed foods are not all bad. Indeed, it would be hard to imagine a modern economy and civilisation without the food processing industry and the supermarket chains that distribute processed food products.

I discovered some interesting facts about food processing on the internet.

Development of food processing
Food processing dates back to our pre-history ... when fire was discovered and cooking invented. The various ways in which food can be cooked are all forms of food processing.

Food preservation also began in pre-history, and the first 'long shelf-life' foods were produced by drying food in the sun and by preserving food with salt. Preservation with salt was common with soldiers, sailors and other travellers until canning was invented in the early 19th century.

One of the first ready-to-eat meals was devised by the ancient Celts when they invented the haggis and what is now known as the Cornish pasty. Another processed food, cheese, is said to have been invented by the nomads of Arabia when they noticed how milk curdled as they jogged along all day on their camels and ponies.

The pre-historic methods of cooking and preserving food remained largely unchanged until the industrial revolution.

The development of modern food processing technology began in the early 19th century in response to the needs of the military. In 1809 a vacuum bottling technique was invented so Napoleon could feed his troops. Canning was invented in 1810 and, after the makers of the cans stopped using lead (which is highly poisonous), canned goods became common throughout the world. Pasteurisation, discovered in 1862, advanced the micro-biological safety of milk and similar products significantly.

Cooling decreases the reproductive rate of bacteria and thus the rate at which food spoils. This storage technique has been in use for hundreds of years. Ice-houses, packed with fresh snow during the winter, were used to preserve food by chilling from the mid-18th century onwards and worked fairly well most of the year round in northern climates.

Commercial refrigeration, using toxic refrigerants which made the technology unsafe in the home, was in use for almost four decades before the first domestic refrigerators were introduced in 1915. In the 1930s, these gained wide acceptance when non-toxic and non-flammable refrigerants such as Freon were invented.

The expansion of the food processing industry later in the 20th century was due to three needs: (a) food to feed the troops efficiently during World War II, (b) food that could be consumed under conditions of zero gravity during forays into outer space, and (c) the pursuit of the convenience demanded by the busy consumer society.

To respond to these needs food scientists invented freeze-drying, spray-drying, and juice concentrates among a host of other processing technologies. They also introduced artificial sweeteners, colouring agents and chemical preservatives. In the closing years of the last century they came up with dried instant soups, reconstituted juices and fruits, and the 'self-cooking' meals (MREs) so beloved of military brass but not the grunts.

The 'pursuit of convenience' has lead to the expansion of frozen foods from simple bags of frozen peas to juice concentrates and complex TV dinners. Those who process food now use the perceived value of time as the foundation of their market appeal.

Benefits
When first produced, processed foods helped to alleviate food shortages and improve overall nutrition by making new foods available globally. Modern food processing delivers many benefits.

By de-activating the pathogenic micro-organisms found in fresh vegetables and raw meats (such as salmonella), processing can reduce food-borne diseases and make food safer.

Because processed foods are less susceptible to spoilage than fresh foods, modern processing, storage and transportation can deliver a wide variety of food from around the world. The choices we have would have been unimaginable to our ancestors.

Processing can often improve the taste of food. It can also have the opposite effect.

The nutritional value of food can be increased by the addition of extra nutrients and vitamins during processing. The nutritional value can also be made more consistent and reliable.

Modern processing technologies can also improve the quality of life for people who have allergies by removing the proteins that cause allergic reactions.

The mass production of food leads to economies of scale for manufacturers. Processed foods are much cheaper to produce than the cost of making meals from raw ingredients in the home.

Processed foods are also extremely convenient. Households are freed from the time-consuming tasks of preparing and cooking foods that are in their natural state ... the food processing industry makes everything from peeled potatoes ready for boiling to prepared-meals that just have to be heated in a micro-wave oven for a few minutes.

Hazards

Processed foods are undoubtedly a great boon. But all is not sweetness and light.

Generally speaking, fresh unprocessed food will contain a higher proportion of naturally occurring fibre, vitamins and minerals than the same food after processing by the food industry. Vitamin C, for example, is destroyed by heat and so fresh fruit will contain more vitamin C than canned fruit.

Indeed, nutrients are often deliberately removed from food during processing in order to improve taste, appearance or shelf-life. Examples include bread, pasta and ready-made meals.

The result is empty calories. Processed foods have a higher ratio of calories to other essential nutrients than fresh, unprocessed foods. They are often energy-dense while being nutritionally poor.

Processing can introduce hazards that are not found in unprocessed foods, due to additives, preservatives, chemically-hardened vegetable oils or trans-fats, and excessive sugar and salt. Indeed, the additives in processed foods ... flavourings, sweeteners, stabilisers, texture-enhancing agents and preservatives among other ... may have little or no nutritive value, or may actually be unhealthy.

Preservatives used to extend shelf-life, such as nitrites or sulphites, may lead to ill-health. In fact, the addition of many chemicals for flavouring and preservation has been shown to cause human and animal cells to grow rapidly, without dying off, thus increasing the risk of a variety of cancers.

Cheap ingredients that mimic the properties of natural ingredients, such as trans-fats made by chemically-hardening vegetable oils that take the place of more-expensive natural saturated fats or cold-pressed oils, have been shown to cause severe health problems in numerous studies. But they are still widely used because of their low-cost and consumer ignorance.

Sugars, fats and salts are usually added to processed foods to improve flavour and as preservatives. As diabetics, we are all well aware of the effects of excessive sugar, fat and on our already damaged systems. Eating large amounts of processed food means consuming too much sugars, fats and salts, which can lead to a variety of health problems such as high blood pressure, cardiovascular diseases, ulcers, stomach cancer, obesity, and diabetes.

Another problem with processed foods is that, where low-quality ingredients are used, this can be disguised during manufacturing.

In the processing industry, a food product will go through several intermediate steps in independent factories before it is finalised in the factory that finishes it.

This is similar to the use of sub-contractors in car manufacturing, where many independent factories products parts, such as electrical systems, bumpers, and other sub-systems, in accordance with the final manufacturer's specifications. These parts are then sold to the car plant where the car is finally assembled from the bought-in parts.

Because the ingredients in processed foods are often made in large quantities during the early stages of the manufacturing process, any hygiene problems in the facilities that produce a basic ingredient that is used widely by other factories in the later stages of production can have serious effects on the quality and safety of many final food products.

Despite the hazards, everyone eats processed foods almost exclusively nowadays. As a result, people eat more quickly and no longer seem aware of the way food is grown and how it is a gift of nature. It seems, also, that food has become more of a necessary interruption in our busy lives and less of a social occasion to be enjoyed.

Eating processed foods

You can't get away from eating some processed foods … the convenience is irresistible.

When you eat processed foods you reduce the likelihood of being poisoned or of picking up a food-borne disease. The nutritional value of what you eat may be more consistent and you will probably be ingesting more nutrients and vitamins than you would get by eating only unprocessed food.

On the other hand, by eating processed foods you are exposing yourself to a potential loss of heat-sensitive vitamins and nutrients that are removed to improve shelf-life, taste and appearance. You are also exposing yourself to the potential adverse effects on your health of various additives and preservatives, some of which can be very serious indeed.

The calorie-dense nature of processed foods, due to the large quantities of sugars and fats they contain, makes them extremely problematic for diabetics and those with high cholesterol and blood pressure levels.

The only solution is to choose the processed foods you buy with extreme care … by reading the labels on the packaging ... and to focus your diet on fresh or frozen produce as much as possible.

12 - Low in Sugar

It may be a truism, but ... eating foods that are low in sugar and that are digested slowly will reduce the amount of, and rate at which, glucose is released into your bloodstream. Doing so is absolutely necessary in order to beat your diabetes.

Sugar can be divided into two groups: (1) sugars that occur naturally in foods such as fruit, and (2) sugar that is added to food and drink by manufacturers.

Manufacturers add sugar (usually refined sugar) during food processing for two good reasons: (a) as a preservative (eg, in jam-making), and (b) to aid fermentation (eg, when making bread).

They also add it for two less worthy reasons: (c) to improve the colour of processed foods and (d) to cater to our sweet teeth.

Most of us have developed extremely sweet teeth which we insist on indulging first thing in the morning. According to Which? Magazine, 76% (152 out of 200) breakfast cereals contain high levels of sugar. Kellogg's Special K (a healthy choice according to its marketing blurb), for instance, contains almost as much sugar as Tesco's Dark Chocolate Fudge Cake Premium Ice Cream.

Is it any wonder that sugar-related diseases such as diabetes are reaching epidemic levels?

Our sweet teeth are acquired very early in life because, as infants and children, we are swamped with sugar. Farleys' Rusks contain more sugar than biscuits such as chocolate digestives (popular biscuits or cookies). Kellogg's Coco Pops and Frosties contain 37% pure sugar per serving.

The problem is that the refined sugar added during food processing contains no nutrients, no vitamins and no fibre. This is the main reason our overall health has deteriorated since we replaced the fruit and vegetables in our diets with sugary foods.

In addition to lacking any nutritional purpose, sugar makes us fat. It is a prime contributor to the obesity that is becoming almost an epidemic in the developed and developing world. A high-sugar diet also raises triglyceride levels which, like cholesterol, clog the arteries and increase our risk of heart attacks and strokes.

Sugary foods also increase the risk that healthy people will develop diabetes. And if you are already a diabetic, too much sugar in your diet results in too much glucose swirling around in your bloodstream and you end up with a series of distressing medical problems as your disease develops.

The dangers of excessive sugar consumption are well-known in the medical world. Indeed, the UN's World Health Organisation (WHO) has recommended that sugar make up no more than 10% of a healthy diet ... this is the figure for healthy people.

As a diabetic, you are better off aiming much lower, as low as possible ... you should minimise your intake of sugar.

However, even if you follow the WHO's recommendation, you will find sticking to the 10% guideline extremely difficult. If your diet gives you 2,000 calories a day, your sugar (at 10%) is limited to just 200 calories ... that is, 50g a day.

But one 500ml bottle of cola contains 50g of sugar. So if you drink one bottle of Coke, you've used up your entire WHO sugar allowance for the day. If you put two teaspoons of sugar in your coffee and drink five cups a day, you've had 40g of sugar (80% of the allowance) before you've even counted the sugar in what you eat.

In addition, it's very hard to know exactly how much sugar you are taking in ... indeed it's practically impossible in my view.

Reducing your intake of sugar
However, you can easily reduce the amount of sugar you eat by avoiding obvious sources, such as chocolate and confectionery. You can also minimise your consumption of processed foods.

But, of course, you have to eat some processed foods. So you need to learn how to check the lists of ingredients on the packages for sugar.

When checking labels, look out for words that end in '-ose', such as sucrose, glucose, dextrose, and maltose, all of which are different forms of sugar. Also check for 'syrups' and 'sweeteners', as well as ingredient such as honey, molasses and cane juice.

Look for the figure in grams for 'carbohydrates Xg of which sugars Yg'. One teaspoon of sugar is 4g, so if you divide the figure for sugars in grams by 4, you can calculate roughly how many teaspoons of sugar a product contains.

Sugar substitutes

If you find giving up sugar difficult, substitutes are available.

You can replace white table sugar in recipes with maple or other syrups and sugarcane juices, all of which taste much sweeter ... this reduces the amount of sugar you take in but only marginally.

Low-calorie sweeteners are used in some manufactured desserts, sweets (candies) and chewing gum. These have about half the calories of regular white sugar (check the labels). There are several no-calories sweeteners you can use in your tea or coffee.

The big disadvantage of substitutes for sugar is that they do not break the sweet tooth habit ... so when the substitutes are not available you'll go back to using sugar. This is why I never used sugar substitutes. Instead I de-acquired my sweet tooth and developed an alternative taste for low sugar.

The fundamental problem with sugar, of course, is that it is addictive.

Sugar addition

In controlled studies, researchers have offered volunteers sugary foods and have recorded how much they ate. At another time, under the same conditions, they have given the same volunteers naloxone intravenously and then offered them the same sugary foods.

Naloxone is a medical drug that is usually used to treat persons who have overdosed on heroin. It prevents the heroin from attaching to receptors in the brain. In sugary food studies, the injections of naloxone caused a significant drop in the desire for sweet foods.

This suggests strongly that sugary foods affect the brain in essentially the same way as heroin and other opiates, though obviously not to the same degree. This mild drug-like effect is most clearly seen in foods that contain both sugar and fat, such as cakes, biscuits (cookies) and full-fat ice cream.

Though it is not an opiate, these experiments show that sugar stimulates the release of opiates within the brain and these opiates, in turn, trigger the release of dopamine which generates feelings of pleasure ... in much the same way as recreational drugs such as alcohol, cocaine, and tobacco.

The craving for sugar goes beyond sugar itself and can appear as a craving for foods that release sugar into the bloodstream quickly (foods with a high GI) such as biscuits, crackers, white bread and potatoes.

So, if you are hooked on sugar, what's the solution?

The best thing to do with a sweet tooth is, in my view, to have it pulled ... in other words you have to get rid of an acquired taste that is harming you health and take up a more benevolent acquired taste in its stead. This is not easy but it is what I did.

My own experience of giving up sugar seems to accord the idea that sugar is addictive. When I was first diagnosed with the pre-diabetes, I tried to give up sugar in my tea and coffee. At that time I was living in Kuwait where food and drink tends to be even more sweetened than in the West.

Tea in the Arab world is served in tiny glass cups (*istikana*) which hold the same volume as a double shot of espresso. One or two heaped teaspoons of white sugar are usually added to this small quantity of tea (depending on whether you want medium or sweet). I rather liked the sticky sweet taste of the tea and giving it up was quite difficult. However but I finally succeeded when I realised that, without the sugar, I could actually taste the tea.

Today I much prefer the unique unsweetened taste of a good tea.

But giving up sugar in my Turkish coffee was a much harder struggle. I adored those little cups of sweet black brew ... they delivered a good pick-me-up kick. Without two spoons of sugar the coffee tasted very bitter. The struggle went on for weeks. Eventually, however, I got used to the bitter taste and much prefer it now. In fact, I cannot stand sugar in coffee nowadays.

The take-away is that it is possible to get of one set of acquired tastes (sweet Arabic tea and sweet Turkish coffee) and acquire other healthier tastes (unsweetened tea and bitter Turkish coffee) ... it just takes perseverance.

If I can do it, you can too.

13 - Low in Fat

Some fat is essential in your diet.

Fat provides you with energy and helps maintain your body temperature, repair your tissues, and protect your internal organs. Fats also transport the fat-soluble vitamins (A, D E and K) around your body. In addition, fatty acids are an important fuel for your heart and skeletal muscles.

The efficacy of my diet is based on the fact that type 2 diabetes is mostly caused by fat blocking the insulin receptors in muscle cells and that you need to unblock those receptors by minimising your intake of fat ... the only way to eliminate the probable basic cause of your diabetes.

According to the authorities I have consulted, a handy rule of thumb is to make sure that you get less than 10% of your energy from fat. However, the type of fat you consume is also important in order to control your levels of cholesterol and triglycerides.

Animal fats are complex mixtures of triglycerides and cholesterol (among other ingredients) and all foods containing animal fat contain cholesterol to varying extents. Plant fat, on the other hand, does not contain any cholesterol.

Thus, avoiding animal fats as far as possible will minimise your intake of cholesterol and reduce the chances of plaques building up inside your arteries and eventually blocking them.

Saturated fat

Saturated fat is present in full-fat dairy products, animal fats, chocolate and several types of oil.

A diet that avoids saturated fats is crucial. To unblock those receptor cells, you must swap the saturated fat found in meats for the mono-unsaturated fat found in plants. And, to reduce your cholesterol levels, you must limit saturated fats to a maximum 7% of your daily intake of calories.

Cholesterol

You can minimise the cholesterol you eat by avoiding foods in which cholesterol is concentrated ... meats high in saturated fat (beef, pork, poultry and shrimp), egg yolks, and whole milk and its products (eg, cheeses).

Though plants contain no cholesterol, foods such as flax seeds and peanuts contain phytosterols. *Phytosterols* are compounds that are similar to cholesterol and some scientists believe that they may help lower cholesterol levels.

In fact, the ideal diet for lowering cholesterol means ... eating no animal products ... minimising your use of vegetable oils ... and eating foods that lower cholesterol (beans, oats, and soy products).

At the same time, you need to lose weight ... each pound you lose lowers your overall cholesterol level by about 1mg/dl. You also need to take up regular exercise ...which will lower your overall cholesterol level, increase your HDL (good) cholesterol, and keep your blood pressure under control.

You HDL levels can be boosted by ... eating beans ... eating fruit and vegetables rich in vitamin C ... avoiding partially-hydrogenated oils ... losing weight ... regular aerobic exercise ... and giving up smoking.

Triglycerides

Cutting back on your calories is crucial in order to reduce triglycerides, because extra calories are converted to triglycerides and stored as fat.

You must also avoid refined and sugary food, because simple carbohydrates (which release glucose into your bloodstream quickly), such as foods made with white floor and sugar, can increase triglycerides.

You can reduce your concentrations of triglycerides by ... eating foods high in fibre ... eating low GI foods (that release glucose slowly) ... eating beans (reduces triglycerides by up to 17%) ... not eating sugar, white bread and related products, and other high GI foods ... not drinking alcohol ... losing weight ... and exercising regularly (eg, walking lowers triglyceride levels by 10mg/dl on average).

Trans-fats

Trans-fats are created artificially for commercial profit by the partial hydrogenation of unsaturated fats. As discussed previously, by increasing LDL (bad) cholesterol and lowering your HDL cholesterol, trans-fats adversely affect your cholesterol ratio. You must eliminate them from your diet.

Trans-fats are found most often in margarine and hydrogenated vegetable fat. You get them from commercial snack foods, fried take-away products, baked products, biscuits (cookies) and crackers.

In some countries foods that contain small quantities of trans-fat can be labelled as 'trans-fat free'; eg, in the USA, a food with less than 0.5g of trans-fat per serving can be trumpeted as 'trans-fat free'. Even though 0.5g is very small, if you eat a lot of that food, the amount can add up quickly.

But how can you know whether a food is completely trans-fat free? The trick is to study the list of ingredients carefully. If it shows 'partially hydrogenated oil', it means the product contains trans-fats, even if only in minute quantities.

Put it back on the shelf and move on.

Foods that lower cholesterol and triglycerides

To beat your diabetes you need to control the overall amount of fat you eat and to minimise your consumption of animal fats. Simply switching from an animal-focused to a plant-focused diet will do the trick.

However, as a type 2 diabetic there is an 85% chance you also have issues with your cholesterol and triglycerides levels. To get these under control you need foods that are effective in lowering your total and LDL ('bad') cholesterol levels, in lowering your triglycerides levels and in raising your HDL levels, and in protecting you from the damage caused by excessive cholesterol and triglycerides.

Happily there seems to be plenty of foods about with these magical qualities … oats, barley and beans…fruits and vegetables … soy … almonds and walnuts … garlic … fruit juices fortified with sterols and stanols … and certain margarines.

Oats, barley and beans contain soluble fibre, which reduces levels of cholesterol and triglycerides.

Eat plenty of beans ... compared to those who don't eat beans at all, people who eat four ounces of beans every day have been found to have overall cholesterol levels that are (on average) 7% lower, LDL cholesterol levels about 6% lower, triglyceride levels averaging 17% lower, and HDL ('good') cholesterol levels about 3% higher ... a true magical food.

Fruits and vegetables are very low in fat, contain soluble fibre and are cholesterol free. Vitamins C and E, and beta-carotene protect the cholesterol particles in your bloodstream from becoming damaged, thus helping to prevent the build-up of plaque on the walls of your arteries. You will find Vitamin C in citrus fruits (oranges, etc) and other fruits and vegetables. Vitamin E turns up in whole grains, vegetables and beans. Beta-carotene is found in orange-coloured vegetables (carrots, pumpkins and yams) and green vegetables.

Soy products, which contain no cholesterol or animal fat, seem to lower levels of cholesterol and triglycerides, though scientists have not yet settled the issue. However, when you do eat soy products you can be sure that you are not taking in any cholesterol.

Almonds and walnuts have an ability to reduce cholesterol levels that is not understood. Like other nuts, they are high in fat ... so you should avoid these nuts (along with all nuts), as the fats they contain may interfere with your efforts to improve your insulin sensitivity.

Garlic may have the ability to lower cholesterol. However not all researchers agree. In studies where garlic has been shown to be effective, at least 1/2 an ounce had to be eaten every day.

Plant sterols and stanols block the absorption of cholesterol from the small intestine. These are natural substances found in many vegetables, but in such small quantities that they have little impact when you eat vegetables.

However, according to researchers, drinking two 8-oz glasses of orange juice fortified with sterols and stanols each day can lower your LDL ('bad') cholesterol by up to 50%, and as high triglyceride levels are associated with high LDL levels, your triglycerides should also be reduced.

A few margarines (eg, Benecol Light) contain natural plant stanols or sterols mixed into a spread made from soybean or canola oil. These margarines can be used in frying or baking. But, as one tablespoon usually contains at least 50 calories, you cannot use them as a low-fat spreads.

Oily fish or supplements containing omega 3 fatty acids are also necessary to control the levels of your cholesterol and triglycerides. However, as you are diabetic, you need to avoid oily fish (because its fat will block the insulin receptors in your cells) and take supplements instead.

14 - Low in Salt

Small quantities of it are essential for life. However, salt is harmful, to diabetics and non-diabetics alike, when taken in excess. Thus, generally speaking, a low salt diet is necessary for your health.

Salt does not affect the levels of your blood glucose. However, high blood pressure can be caused by a high intake of salt and diabetics are much more likely to get hypertension than non-diabetics.

As you have diabetes you have a much higher risk of developing problems relating you heart, nervous system, kidneys and eyes than a non-diabetic. If you are also hypertensive, the risks from both diseases are combined and the likelihood that you will develop coronary artery disease or an enlarged heart is increased yet again.

Table salt (refined salt) contains about 97% to 99% sodium chloride. Thus table salt has about 40% sodium and 60% chloride by weight. It is the sodium in salt that contributes to high blood pressure.

Function of salt

Salt is vital for optimal bodily function.

Sodium in involved in ... regulating the water content (fluid balance) of the body ... maintaining the acid-base balance ... transmitting nerve impulses ... regulating muscle contractions, and ... absorbing and transporting some nutrients.

However, too much salt increases the risk of health problems, including ... stroke and cardiovascular disease ... hypertension (high blood pressure) ... left ventricular hypertrophy (enlargement of the heart) ... oedema (fluid retention) ... duodenal ulcers and gastric ulcers, and ... heartburn.

A large-scale study published in 2007 indicated that people who reduced the amount of salt in their diet decreased their risk of developing cardiovascular disease by 25% over the following 10 to 15 years and their risk of dying from cardiovascular disease by 20%.

However the consequences of eating too little or too much salt vary from person to person, and a few scientists have asserted that the risks from consuming too much salt have been exaggerated for most people or that the studies on the consumption of salt are open to various interpretations.

Doctors cannot tell whether is a person is sodium sensitive or likely to develop high blood pressure from consuming too much salt. Nevertheless, many medical scientists are of the opinion that if we all permanently reduced our salt intakes by modest amounts, the long-term result would be lower blood pressure and fewer strokes and heart attacks among the population as a whole.

Recommended intake

The recommended daily intake of salt and sodium varies from country to country and there seems to be no consensus on the issue. Indeed, when I checked the recommended intakes according to official sources in several Western countries I was astounded at the range of opinions.

An adequate intake ranges from 1.15–2.3g of salt (0.46–0.92g of sodium) a day, according to the National Health & Medical Research Council (NHMRC) in Australia, to 3–3.75g of salt (1.2–1.5g of sodium) a day, according to Health Canada.

This means that the recommended daily intake in Canada is more than two-and-a-half times the recommended intake in Australia. It's obvious that the effects of salt and sodium in the diet are not understood by medical scientists.

According to the NHMRC in Australia and the USA's Dietary Guidelines for Americans 2010, the recommended upper limit is 5.75g of salt (2.3g of sodium), about one somewhat-heaped teaspoon of salt. These are upper limits are just that ... upper limits ... and are not your optimal intake.

All health authorities seem to agree that some people are especially sensitive to the harmful effects of salt ... people with diabetes, hypertension and chronic kidney disease, and the elderly ... and that the intake for such people should be much lower than for other adults, typically one-third less.

The problem is that most adults (healthy and not so healthy) are consuming 4 to 6g of sodium daily, ie most of us are ingesting at least double the upper limits recommended by most health authorities.

The American Dietary Guidelines provide a Dietary Reference Intake for sodium showing what your salt intake per day (for healthy persons) should be at different ages:

- 1.5mg sodium (3.75g salt) – 19-50 years of age
- 1.3mg sodium (3.25g salt) – 51-70 years of age
- 1.2mg sodium (3.00g salt) – over 71 years of age

My personal view is that these limits are a bit high. Increased total body sodium and enhanced vascular reactivity have been found in people with diabetes and most type 2 diabetic patients are sensitive to salt. A high salt diet in type 2 diabetics who are also hypertensive has been associated with a reduced volume of blood being delivered to the kidneys.

Thus, I try to limit my salt intake to the amounts recommended by the NHMRC in Australia as adequate: 1.15–2.3g of salt (0.46–0.92g of sodium) a day. It's not too difficult.

Sources of sodium
Our intake of sodium comes from six main sources ... processed foods ... cooking ... the salt-shaker ... unprocessed foods ... drinking water ... and medications.

Processed foods provide most of the sodium in our diets. Salt or other sodium compounds are added during processing either to enhance flavour or as preservatives.

These other sodium compounds include additives such as ... monosodium glutamate (MSG, a flavour enhancer) ... disodium phosphate (to speed up the cooking time of 'quick cook' cereals) ... sodium alginate (to hold chocolate in suspension in milk and ice cream) ... sodium benzoate (a preservative) ... and sodium propionate (a preservative that inhibits mould in bread and cakes).

Some of these added compounds are bizarre. Sodium hydroxide (aka lye or caustic soda), which is used for washing and chemical peeling, is also used to process chocolate and cocoa, to thicken ice cream and as a glaze in baking. Ugh!

Processed foods include cured meats (eg, bacon, sausages, hot dogs, bologna), pickled food (pickles, sauerkraut, olives etc), some canned vegetables (such as peas and beans), many snack foods (potato crisps, corn chips, crackers etc), packaged sauces (including soy sauce). The sodium content should be shown on the labelling.

A level teaspoon of salt contains about 2g of sodium, at least double the amount I personally would wish to ingest each day. For this reason I seldom add salt during cooking and never use the salt-shaker over my food.

Unprocessed foods are not sodium-free. All fresh-meat and fish contain some sodium as do all plants. Some vegetables contain more sodium than others, eg, carrots, spinach, celery and beet.

Drinking water also contains sodium. However soft water contains more than hard water and water softeners increase the sodium content. The amount of sodium varies from region to region. The sodium content should be shown on the labelling for bottled water.

Many over-the-counter medications contain sodium. These include headache and indigestion tablets, laxatives and cough medicines. The sodium content is shown on the labelling.

Labelling

The labelling requirements for foods containing salt and sodium vary from country to country, but generally speaking, most countries require the amount of salt and/or sodium in either 100g or in a single 'serving' to be stated on the label. Sometimes both are required.

However, the requirements for descriptive words or phrases relating to low sodium content vary markedly.

In the USA, the FDA *Food Labelling Guide* stipulates that ... *sodium free* means 5mg or less per serving ... *very low sodium* means 35mg or less per serving ... and *low sodium* means 140mg or less per serving.

In addition, a product can only be described as *reduced sodium* if the usual levels of sodium have been reduced by at least 25 percent. And it can only be described as *unsalted* or *no salt added* if no salt was added during processing (which does not necessarily mean that it is salt-free, just that no salt was added).

The American regulations also stipulate that, when other health claims are being made about a food (eg, that it is low in fat or calories), the amount of sodium must be shown where the food contains more than 0.48g per serving.

In the UK, the Food Standards Agency defines the level of salt in foods as follows ... high means more than 1.5g salt (0.6 g sodium) per 100g of food ... low means 0.3g salt (or 0.1 g sodium) or less per 100g ... and medium is an amount in between these figures.

Just checking the salt content on a label may not be enough. You also need to check the label for monosodium glutamate and the other additives mentioned above.

Eating less salt

To reduce your daily intake of sodium, you need to avoid foods that are high in salt. This is the best thing to do ... and it's dead easy.

Some people use substitutes in which sodium is replaced with other components. These substitutes contain mostly potassium chloride, which increases potassium intake. Increasing potassium intake shouldn't be a problem for a healthy adult.

However various diseases and medications can reduce the body's excretion of potassium and excess potassium intake can cause your heart to beat abnormally. Thus, those who have diabetes or heart or kidney problems should seek medical advice before using a salt substitute.

Personally I'm against using a salt substitute. If you are in the habit of grabbing the salt-shaker to flavour your food, use herbs or spices as condiments instead.

You can also reduce the salt in your diet by buying less salty foods. Just check the food labels on the packages for the sodium content.

Most Westerners get about three-quarters of the salt they ingest from pre-prepared and processed foods, so a good strategy would be to reduce these as much as possible. With modern labelling standards, you should have no problem in choosing low-sodium or salt-free items.

You can also reduce the sodium in your diet by switching the kinds of food you eat. Instead of cured, smoked or canned meats, go for fresh fish, poultry or beef. Opt for fresh fruit and vegetables instead of tinned (canned) varieties with additives. Whole-grain foods such as wheat bread, pasta and brown rice are lower in sodium than the usual varieties.

One of the great truths I discovered while researching how to beat diabetes is that all our tastes ... with the exception of mother's milk ... are acquired tastes. What is acquired can be de-acquired ... it's just a matter of retraining your palate.

I also found that there's nothing easier than reducing the amount of salt and sodium in your diet. Once you've dropped the habit of salt-with-everything, you'll find that your taste-buds are becoming quite sensitive to salt and it'll be easier to avoid. At least, that's what I discovered.

15 - High in Fibre

It was once called roughage. As kids, whenever we got a bit constipated, the solution was to 'eat more roughage'.

I used to have visions of vast quantities of stalks that had to be consumed as a sort of punishment for getting bunged up … and, indeed, 'more roughage' usually came in the form of celery and other plants that required a fair bit of chewing.

In fact, *dietary fibre* is the indigestible portion of plant foods. And, there are two types of dietary fibre. Both kinds are highly beneficial and eating plenty of them is crucial for beating diabetes.

Soluble fibre is fibre that dissolves in water to form a viscous gel-like material. It is fermented by bacteria in the digestive tract and changes how other nutrients and chemicals are absorbed. It lowers your levels of blood glucose, LDL ('bad') cholesterol and triglycerides.

Insoluble fibre cannot dissolve in water. It merely passes through your system. It absorbs water, however, and makes your stool more bulky. This eases defecation which makes constipation less likely.

Both types of fibre are absolutely necessary for a healthy diet. All plants contain some fibre, of both kinds, to a greater or lesser degree. The overall quantity and the relative amounts of soluble and insoluble fibre vary from species to species.

The main sources of soluble fibre are … legumes (beans, peas, etc) … grains such as oats, rye and barley … vegetables such as broccoli, carrot and artichokes … root vegetables such as sweet potatoes and onions … and the insides of some fruits (and therefore their juices) such as prunes, plums, berries, bananas, apples and pears.

Insoluble fibre is mostly found in … whole grains … wheat and corn bran … nuts and seeds … potato skins … flax seeds … fruit such as avocados and bananas … some skins such as on tomatoes … and vegetables such as green beans, cauliflower, courgettes (zucchini) and celery.

Some plants contain significant amounts of both soluble and insoluble fibre. The juicy pulp inside a plum, for instance, contains lots of soluble fibre, while the outside skin is full of insoluble fibre.

Other plants that contain both types include sweet potatoes, onions, apples, pears, berries and prunes.

Benefits of dietary fibre

To beat diabetes, you have to control the levels of your blood glucose, cholesterol and triglycerides, and your blood pressure. Dietary fibre helps immensely in this battle. Here's what I found out through internet research.

Rapid satiety ... high-fibre food is less energy-dense than other food ... it contains fewer calories than the same volume of food with less fibre.

This means that you are less likely to over-eat as high-fibre food makes you feel full quicker. The bulkiness of high-fibre meals also tends to keep you satiated for longer, thus helping you control your weight, another essential for beating your diabetes.

Glucose ... food high in soluble fibre slows the absorption of sugar. This is because, when it dissolves and turns to a gel during digestion, it traps carbohydrates and stabilizes the release of insulin from the pancreas.

Slowing the rate at which glucose is released reduces its peak concentrations in your bloodstream. You can exploit this immensely handy fact to control your blood glucose levels.

Cholesterol: the soluble fibre found in beans, oats, flax-seed and oat-bran suppresses the synthesis of cholesterol by the liver.

This reduces your levels of LDL ('bad') cholesterol and triglycerides and can be significant factor in beating your diabetes by keeping your cholesterol levels under control.

Blood pressure: some studies have shown that increasing fibre in the diet reduces blood pressure.

Bowel movements: dietary fibre increases the weight and size of your stool and softens it. A bulky stool is easier to pass.

High-fibre diets make it less likely that you will suffer from constipation, provided you drink plenty of water with your meals. Because it absorbs water and adds bulk, fibre can also help to solidify loose, watery stools.

Bowel health: by making your stool easier and therefore quicker to pass, high-fibre diets lower your risk of developing haemorrhoids and diverticulitis (in which small pouches in your colon become inflamed and infected, a very painful condition with which I am thoroughly familiar), provided you complement your high-fibre diet with plenty of plain water.

Many other benefits have been associated with high-fibre diets. The fermentation of fibre in the colon, for example, may reduce the risk of colorectal cancer and other diseases of the colon.

Dietary fibre does not bind to vitamins and minerals and therefore it does not inhibit their absorption. Indeed, some research shows that fermentable soluble fibre improves the absorption of some minerals such as calcium.

Water

To gain the full benefits of a high-fibre diet, you must drink plenty of water.

This is absolutely necessary so that you have sufficient water to dissolve all the soluble fibre you eat, with plenty left over to lubricate the passage of insoluble fibre through your digestive system ... overall, at least 2 litres a day on top of all the other liquids (tea, coffee, juices, etc) you drink. That's what I do.

Healthy quantities

The big question is ... how much dietary fibre should you ingest daily?

In the view of medical scientists, the simple answer is ... at least 40gm a day, along with plenty of water.

However, official recommendations are often much lower. For example, the Institute of Medicine, a non-governmental organisation (NGO) which is part of the US National Academy of Sciences, recommends that adults should consume 20 to 35 grams of dietary fibre a day.

The American Diabetes Association also recommends 20 to 35 grams a day as a minimum for healthy adults but states that the actual amount consumed should vary within these limits according to a person's daily calorie intake. For example, the ADA recommends that a person who eats 2,000 calories a day should include 25g of fibre in their daily diet.

These recommendations however are for healthy adults. I have discovered that the upper limit of 35g a day is considered somewhat low by medical scientists who are researching ways of beating diabetes and heart diseases using diet alone or diet in combination with exercise programmes.

The consensus of these researchers is that the minimum intake of dietary fibre for persons with diabetes, and related conditions such as cardiovascular problems, is 40 grams a day ... along with plenty of water throughout the day.

Figuring out what foods and how much of them you need to eat to achieve a fibre intake of 40g a day sounds complicated. It is not ... in fact, nothing could be easier.

Ready-reckoner
To find out how much fibre you are eating, you need to list everything you eat or drink for one day, along with the quantity (ie number of servings) of each of these foods. You then multiply the various quantities by the number of grams of fibre in a serving for those particular foods.

Sounds complicated? It isn't ... it's a cinch.

On www.beating-diabetes.com you will find a handy form you can download and use to list the foods and quantities you eat, as well as a chart showing the number of grams of fibre in a serving for an individual food, along with easy-to-follow instructions. Just click on *Signup and download Checklists & References* under DOWNLOADS.

The form has three columns, one for each particular food item, another for the quantity, and a final column for that food's 'fibre score'.

All you have to do is list each food item and put the quantity next to it. Then you work out the fibre-score by multiplying each quantity by the appropriate number of grams as shown on the chart. After that, just add up the fibre-scores for each item to get the total amount of fibre you ate that day.

If you score:

- Less than 20g ... you are not getting enough fibre and need to up

your intake greatly
- 20 - 39g ... you're doing better than most Westerners but still need to increase your intake
- 40g or over ... you are on target

Doing this quick check is pretty simple and only takes a few minutes. The benefit is that it will give you a rough idea as to whether or not you are getting enough fibre in your diet. If you can get your total daily figure up to more than forty, you can be sure that you are eating all the fibre you need. If it's well over 40, don't worry ... you can't over-eat fibre!

Don't worry either about the proportions of soluble and insoluble fibre in your diet. As long as you eat a good mix of vegetables, fruit, and grains the balance will take care of itself automatically.

You only need to use the ready-reckoner once a week at first. Once you are up to 40 grams a day, there is no need to do the check. As long as you stay on course eating a high-fibre diet, checking every few months or so would be sufficient.

I found this ready-reckoner (which I cribbed from Dr Neal Barnard's *Program for Reversing Diabetes*) very useful when I was first trying to up my intake of fibre. Now that I'm pretty much up to speed on dietary fibre and know how much I can get from all sorts of food products, I don't bother with it much anymore, just an occasional check once or twice a year.

The ready-reckoner does not include a scoring mechanism for processed food products. This is because the fibre content will be displayed on the packaging, a legal requirement in most countries. Just estimate the amount you have eaten and then use the details from the packaging to figure out how much fibre you have ingested and add the number in at the bottom of the form.

Processed food products
Processed foods ... such as some canned fruits and vegetables, pulp-free juices, white bread, some pastas, and cereals made from refined grains ... have less fibre content than natural foods.

This is because the skins are often removed when fruit and vegetables are being canned. When grains are refined, the fibrous bran (outer coating) is removed. Indeed, most forms of processing remove the fibre content of fruit and vegetables.

Nevertheless, many of the processed commercial foodstuffs you buy in supermarkets do contain some fibre ... read the labels.

However I do feel that getting your fibre from natural unaltered sources (fresh fruit and vegetables) is superior for beating diabetes, and this is what I try to do myself as much as possible.

Fibre supplements

There are plenty of fibre supplements around. These are marketed as aids for improving nutrition, for treating various gastro-intestinal disorders, for lowering cholesterol levels, reducing the risk of colon cancer, for losing weight, and so on.

The hype is phenomenal. In my view, fibre supplements may be warranted if you suffer from serious medical conditions, such as constipation, diarrhoea or irritable bowel syndrome. If so, you should follow your doctor's advice and take whatever fibre supplements he or she suggests.

But which is better ... swallowing a pill ... or enjoying a nice juicy piece of fruit? When you choose the fruit, you also get the all the other beneficial nutrients, vitamins and minerals a fruit contains, along with the fibre you need to beat your diabetes.

So I feel that you should forget about fibre supplements unless your doctor prescribes otherwise.

16 – Low Glycemic Index Values

During the digestive process, some types of food release glucose into your bloodstream at faster rates than others.

Consider bread and pasta.

When bread is made, yeast is added to lighten it and make it easier to eat. The yeast causes tiny pockets of air to form in the flour and the dough rises. When you eat bread your digestive juices can enter these air-pockets easily, where they can break down the molecules of flour into molecules of glucose very quickly. The glucose then passes through your digestive tract into your bloodstream.

Pasta is different. Though it is also made from wheat, no yeast is added to the flour and so it has no pockets of air. Provided it has not been overcooked, pasta cannot be digested as quickly as bread. Thus it releases glucose into your bloodstream at a much slower rate than bread.

Again, a heavily processed grain, such as quick-cooking oatmeal (in which the grains have been pulverised into flour), will start to come apart in your stomach quickly ... while an intact grain, such as whole oats, will break down and release glucose into your bloodstream much more slowly.

The implications for controlling the level of glucose in the bloodstream are obvious. By slowing down the release of glucose, you reduce your demand for insulin and less insulin is released into your bloodstream.

Indeed, in the opinion of many medical scientists, foods that release glucose slowly improve the long-term control of blood glucose levels. These are the foods diabetics should eat.

The question is ... how do you know which foods are 'slow-release' foods?

Answer ... you consult the glycemic index (GI) which ranks various foods according to how quickly they break-down in the stomach and release glucose into the bloodstream.

The GI values of specific foods are determined by nutritional scientists under laboratory conditions. They are then published and made widely available.

Determining GI values

The GI value of a particular food (spaghetti, say) is determined by feeding 10 healthy adults (who have been fasting overnight) a serving that contains 50 grams of digestible carbohydrate.

Their blood glucose levels are measured just before they eat and at 15 minute intervals over the following two hours and the results are plotted on individual graphs.

A typical graph shows a curve that rises, as glucose is released into the bloodstream, to a peak and then falls off as the glucose leaves the bloodstream either by being ushered into the muscle cells by insulin or by exiting into the kidneys whence it is excreted via the urine.

Following another overnight fast, the same 10 people are each given a syrup containing 50 grams of glucose (the reference food). Their blood glucose levels are measured as before and the individual results plotted.

For each of the 10 adults, the GI value of the test-food is calculated by comparing the glucose values for the food with the results from the reference food using advanced mathematical techniques. The final GI value of the test-food is the average of the GI values obtained from each participant.

By giving the reference food a GI value of 100, the average GI values of particular foods can be ranked ... on a scale of 1 to 100 ... according to their relationships to the reference food.

For instance, yam has a GI value of 51, which means that it releases glucose into your bloodstream much more slowly than the reference food, while baked potato has a GI value of 94, that is, it releases glucose into your bloodstream almost as quickly as the reference food.

Foods with a high GI score contain carbohydrates that are digested rapidly, producing a large, quick rise and fall in blood glucose. The rapid rise in blood glucose makes these the best for getting energy back after strenuous exercise or after abnormal drop in blood glucose (hypoglycaemia).

Foods with a low GI contain carbohydrates that are digested slowly and deliver a smaller and more gradual rise in blood glucose and a slower fall-off. These are the foods diabetics need to eat.

Which foods?

The GI values of various foods can be found at www.glycemicindex.com. You will also find a handy table of GI values at www.beating-diabetes.com which you can download as a PDF file for reference by clicking on *Signup and download Checklists & References* under DOWNLOADS.

Most nutritionists classify GI values as low (up to 55), medium (56–69) or high (70 and greater). The classification is a bit arbitrary but, when you check out lists of foods ranked by their GI values (see the table in *Checklists & References* mentioned in the last paragraph) you will notice that the foods in the low-GI range are mainly plants of various kinds.

Indeed, most fruits and vegetables, pulses (beans, peas, chickpeas and lentils), and whole grains have low GIs. This makes them (with certain exceptions) ideal for diabetics and justifies a plant-based diet as being the most suitable for us.

Note the following:

Fruits ... nearly all fruits have low GI values and, although they are sweet, they do not release glucose into the bloodstream quickly, except for watermelon and pineapple which have quite high GIs.

Bread ... rye breads, such as pumpernickel, have low GIs, but white breads and bagels have relatively high GIs.

Be careful with whole-meal breads. Even though high-fibre unrefined breads have lower GI values than white breads, many types of whole-wheat bread are treated with enzymes to soften the crust which makes the carbohydrates more accessible, so they can have high GI values.

Grains ... most grains are low GI. Pasta is a low-GI food. Barley, bulgur and some types of rice are also low-GI foods. Among the cereals, oatmeal and bran have lower GI values, while most of the breakfast cereals that you eat cold (corn flakes and so on) have higher GI values.

Potatoes ... yams and sweet potatoes are low-GI foods, but ordinary potatoes have higher GI values.

Nuts ... most nuts are also low GI but many are high in fat so they are not suitable for diabetics.

Drawbacks of GI numbers

The glycemic index can only be calculated for foods that contain a reasonable amount of sugar or starch, because the test requires participants to eat enough of the test-food to yield 50g of carbohydrate.

Several berry-type fruits and green-leafy vegetables, such as broccoli and cauliflower, are very high in dietary fibre but contain very little starch. The average person would find it almost impossible to eat enough of these to ingest 50g of carbohydrate, so their GI values cannot be calculated.

Other foods are high in fat and low in starch and so GI numbers cannot be calculated for these foods either. Some protein-heavy foods, such as very lean meats, contain no carbohydrates and therefore have no GI value.

GI food lists are rough approximations only, and any list represents typical, not precise, GI values. This is because the actual GI number obtained for a particular food (apples, say) will vary depending on its variety, ripeness, processing, storage time, cooking methods and other factors. For instance, the GI value for white potatoes can range from moderate to very high even within the same variety.

Determining GI values is, in fact, fairly imprecise for several other significant reasons. The first of these is the fact that the glycemic response of individuals to food varies from person to person. This is due to factors such as differing levels of insulin resistance, and so on.

The GI also fails to take the quantity of a particular food that is eaten into account. Your digestive juices begin breaking down all the carbohydrates in the food you are eating as soon as you swallow.

For example, if you eat 50 grams of a food with a particular carbohydrate content and GI number, you will get a particular glucose curve in your blood. It seems reasonable to assume that if you eat only 25 grams of the same food, you will get a glucose curve with a similar shape except that it will peak will be at half the height, as you will have less glucose in your bloodstream.

The GI of a food is determined after an overnight fast. However, food eaten later in the day can show a different glycemic response than food eaten at breakfast time. Research has shown that when the same food (a standard high-GI breakfast cereal, for example) is eaten twice in equal amounts, with a break of a few hours between each meal, the increase in blood glucose levels is less after the second meal.

It seems that the composition of the first meal can have a strong influence on the glycemic response to the second meal, though the reason is unknown.

In addition, the helpfulness of GI values in beating diabetes is open to question. This is because the glycemic index does not take into account insulin response, the amount of insulin released into your bloodstream when you eat different foods. Insulin response can have a significant effect on your blood glucose levels, but knowing it is not crucial for beating your diabetes.

Not all foods with low GIs will help you beat your diabetes. Some foods that are unhealthy (very often because of their fat content) have a low GI value; chocolate cake (GI 38) and ice cream (GI 37) for instance. So, using GI numbers when choosing what to eat has to be coupled with common sense!

Nevertheless, despite the imprecision of GI values and their short-comings, eating low GI foods has been proven by medical research to bestow significant benefits.

Benefits

If you get at least 50% of your calories from carbohydrates, the glycemic index can enable you to consume the same number of calories and, at the same time, achieve more stable glucose and insulin levels … by indicating, however imprecisely, the foods that are best for you as a diabetic.

Switching to eating mainly low GI carbohydrates that slowly trickle glucose into your blood stream will keep your energy levels balanced. This means that your hunger will be reduced, you will feel full for longer between meals, and your physical endurance will be prolonged.

For a diabetic, a low GI diet (a) increases the body's sensitivity to insulin, (b) improves blood cholesterol levels, (c) helps maintain a healthy weight, and (d) reduces the risk of heart disease.

Thus, eating low-GI food enables you to optimise the management of your diabetes … which is why I have it as an integral part of how I choose the foods to eat.

Glycemic load

One of the drawbacks of the glycemic index is that it does not take quantity into account. The glycemic load (GL) is designed to do that ... by combining the quality (GI value) of a particular food and the amount of carbohydrates (by weight) it contains into one number.

The formula for calculating the GL is very simple. The GL of a particular food is its GI value multiplied by its carbohydrate content as a percentage of its total weight.

For example, watermelon (which is mostly water) has a GI of 72 and contains 5% carbohydrates by weight, so its GL is 72x5/100 = 3.6.

Since the peak reached by the concentration of glucose in your blood is probably the most important thing you have to control when managing your diabetes, multiplying the quantity of carbohydrates in a serving by the glycemic index gives you an idea as to how that portion of a particular food will affect your glucose level.

Like the GI, the GL has a scale and glycemic loads are classified as low (up to 10), medium (11 – 19) and high (20 or more).

As calculated above, watermelons have a GL of 3.6, which is low.

Other examples:

- Carrots have a GL of 3.5 (GI 47x7.5%) which is also low.
- Bananas have a GL of 10.0 (GI 52x20%) which is on the upper limit of low
- Corn tortillas (Mexican) have a GL of 25.0 (GI 52x48%) which is high
- White rice (boiled) has a GL of 15.4 (GI 64x24%) which is medium

While the glycemic load can be useful in enabling you to choose between various low GI products, other than that it is unlikely to be much practical benefit.

Insulin index

Insulin response refers to the amount of insulin that is released into your bloodstream when you eat a particular food. It too can have a crucial effect on your blood glucose levels.

Insulin response is measured using an insulin index (II), which is based on the behaviour of blood insulin levels following the eating of particular foods. The II is calculated in a similar way as the glycemic index, except that white bread is used as the reference food instead of glucose syrup.

The conventional and approved method of calculating the glycemic index is to use glucose syrup as the reference food. This has the advantage that the reference food has a stable, verifiable and precisely defined glucose content, which has a GI value of 100 by definition.

The GI can also be calculated using white bread as the reference food. Doing so results in a different set of GI values, as the reference food is given a value of 100. If white bread had a GI value of 100 then glucose would have a GI value of about 140. The disadvantage of using white bread is that the reference food is not defined very precisely.

However, using white bread as the reference food for calculating GI means that the GI values of various foods can be compared directly with the insulin index (II) of these foods.

The results, when this is done, are very revealing.

Researchers have found that the glucose and insulin scores of most foods are highly correlated, that is they march step-in-step. For these foods, therefore, calculating the II does not make a significant contribution to your ability to control your glucose levels.

However, high protein foods (such as lean meats) and bakery products that are full of refined carbohydrates and fat trigger insulin responses that are much higher than their glycemic responses. For this reason, researchers have concluded that using the II may be useful in managing diets to beat diabetes.

In my view, this is a bit over the top. Worrying about the insulin index (which is still in the process of development, according to my research) will deliver a poor return on your efforts to manage your diabetes. To avoid an excessive insulin response to the foods you eat, all you have to do is ... reduce your consumption of meat proteins to a minimum ... eat only low-fat foods, and ... avoid bakery products such as cakes and confectionary (which you will do instinctively when you check the sugar and fat levels shown on the labels!)

Conclusion

The purpose of the glycemic index is to rate individual foods against each other regarding the speed at which they release glucose into the bloodstream. For persons with type 2 diabetes, ie who have insulin resistance, foods with relatively low GI values, are the most preferable.

In my view, there is no way (without a lot of bother) you can get up to speed on the glycemic load and insulin index. But if you stick to a plant-based diet, most of the food you eat will have low GIs, low GLs and a reasonable insulin response.

In addition, as your digestive system begins breaking down all the carbohydrates in your food as soon as you eat it, you also need to eat not more than a reasonable quantity at any one sitting. That is, as a diabetic, you should eat smaller meals than a 'normal' person but have more meals in a day.

Globally, there are only a few research groups that provide a legitimate testing and certification service for commercial food products. When choosing food products, make sure that any GI symbols on the packaging have been issued by an approved testing laboratory.

17 - Nutritional Supplements

Nutritional supplements can make up for many deficiencies in your diet. However, in extreme cases, certain supplements can be harmful to your health if you take too much of them.

The term *nutritional supplement* covers micro-nutrients such as vitamins, minerals and fatty acids. I feel that spices can also be included where they do more than just enhance flavours.

I was never much of a believer in vitamins and minerals ... until fairly recently.

A few years ago walking was becoming increasingly difficult for me. Due to my diabetic neuropathy, which was slowly getting worse, I could only go a short distance before the soles of my feet began hurting. I could envisage a time when it would get so bad that I would not be able to walk at all. This was before I had started the diet I am following to beat my diabetes.

My brother, a well-known neurologist in the USA, suggested that I try vitamin B12 as a supplement. Despite my initial scepticism, I began taking 4 micrograms (mcg), once in the morning and again at night, twice the recommended daily allowance (RDA).

The effect was dramatic. Within a few days my feet were no longer hurting when I walked. I cut back to the RDA of 4mcg a day. I still take that amount of B12 every day.

Once I was a firm believer in the value of nutritional supplements I began researching the matter extensively on the internet. I have arrived at two overall conclusions:

(a) The functions of all vitamins and minerals are not yet fully understood by scientists, and
(b) The results of clinical tests often contradict each other.

Nevertheless I remain firmly convinced that supplements are necessary to beat your diabetes.

The Office of Dietary Supplements in the National Institutes of Health in the USA issues bulletins detailing the amounts of particular supplement you need every day to ensure good health. These are known as recommended daily allowances (RDAs).

The RDAs for individual substances may vary depending on your age and gender. The American RDAs are accepted as valid by most countries.

The main difference between vitamins and nutritional minerals is that vitamins are organic (ie, they contain carbon) and minerals are inorganic.

Vitamins

Vitamins are vital for health and you need more than a dozen different types ... all of them are different and you cannot substitute one for another. However, some vitamins have several closely-related forms, so what is essentially one vitamin may have several different names.

All vitamins fall into one of two main groups ... water-soluble or fat-soluble.

Water-soluble ... are all the B vitamins plus vitamin C. These vitamins are not stored in your body. When you eat more than you need for immediate use you get rid of the excess in your urine.

Thus the water-soluble vitamins cannot build up to toxic levels in your body and you have to get fresh supplies into your system every day. These vitamins can be included in your daily supplements, just in case you are not getting enough in your food, without any risk of toxicity.

Fat-soluble ... are vitamins A, D, E and K. You need a small amount of fat in your diet in order to absorb these vitamins.

If you eat more than you need immediately, the extra vitamins are stored in your body fat, which means that they could build up to toxic levels in your body. However this is extremely rare.

You don't have to get fresh supplies of fat-soluble vitamins into your system every day, and they are not usually washed out into cooking water (unlike water-soluble vitamins).

Sources of vitamins

Most foods contain a variety of vitamins. But no one food has enough of all of the vitamins to meet your total requirements. Here's an overview of what I found out:

(1) Grains provide four B vitamins: thiamine (B1), riboflavin (B2) niacin (B3), and folate (B9)

(2) Vegetables supply folate (B9), vitamin A, vitamin C and vitamin E, while beans and legumes also provide thiamine (B1).

(3) Fruits give you folate (B9), vitamin A and vitamin C.

(4) Dairy products provide riboflavin (B2), vitamin B12, and (if fortified) vitamins A and D.

(5) Meats and fish provide niacin (B3), thiamine (B1), vitamin B6 and vitamin B12.

(6) Oils provide vitamin E.

All the vitamins you need can be delivered in a low-fat diet. However a plant-focused diet is more problematic ... it will deliver plenty of water-soluble vitamins.

But the main food sources of vitamin D are egg yolk and fish oil, while vitamin E is found in vegetable oils and nuts, especially almonds. Thus, if you follow the sort of diet I use to beat diabetes you will need to take vitamin supplements to get all you need of these vitamins.

This is perfectly OK ... you may not realise it but you are already taking nutritional substances.

Many of the food products you buy in your supermarket are 'fortified' or 'enriched', ie they contain added vitamins and minerals. Vitamin D is usually added to milk to prevent rickets, while niacin (B3) and thiamine (B1) are added to refined flour, corn meal and rice to prevent diseases such as pellagra and beriberi. Thus you are already getting supplements by eating commercially prepared food products.

Minerals

Minerals are divided into two groups ... major minerals and trace minerals.

Major minerals are the minerals you need in amounts of 100 milligrams (mg) or more each day. These minerals are calcium, phosphorus, magnesium, sulphur, potassium, sodium, and chloride.

Trace minerals are needed in amounts of less than 100mg each day. Trace minerals include iron, iodine, zinc, fluoride, selenium, copper, chromium, manganese, and molybdenum.

Minerals are inactive but are used in a variety of processes. For example, your body uses calcium to make bones and teeth, and iron to make the haemoglobin in your red blood cells.

Minerals help to regulate processes such as enzyme systems. They have a role in the transmission of nerve impulses and the contraction of muscles. Minerals also help release energy from food.

The minerals in our food come from a variety of sources:

(1) Grains deliver iron, copper, zinc, manganese, magnesium, molybdenum, chromium, and phosphorus.
(2) Fruit contains magnesium, manganese, and potassium, while vegetables are full of potassium, magnesium, iodine, and selenium.
(3) Meat, eggs and fish provide iron, copper, zinc, chromium, magnesium, potassium, phosphorus, and sulphur.
(4) Dairy products provide calcium, magnesium, phosphorus, and potassium.

If you follow my diet for beating diabetes, you will not be eating any eggs or dairy products and will therefore need to take several minerals in supplemental form.

Other supplements
There are several other dietary supplements which are not, strictly speaking, vitamins or minerals.

Cinnamon ... this spice works wonders for glucose levels. I discovered that it is known to cut fasting glucose levels by up to 30% and helps to reduce cholesterol levels.

To test its effect on glucose levels I began sprinkling it on my porridge (oatmeal) every morning. Within a few days, my average glucose levels first thing in the morning had dropped by nearly 0.5mmol/l (9mg/l).

Cod-liver oil ... my diet to beat diabetes means eating reduced amounts of animal protein and avoiding animal oils as far as possible. Animal in this context covers all fauna including fish. For this reason I take a daily dose of cod-liver oil in a capsule.

Alpha-lipoic acid (thioctic acid) ... is a cofactor for several enzymes involved in energy metabolism.

A *cofactor* is a 'helper' molecule that is needed to assist an enzyme or other protein in its biological activity. Alpha-lipoic acid plays an important role in the mitochondria, the tiny furnaces in the cells that turn fat into energy.

Because the body produces enough alpha-lipoic acid itself, a supplement is not needed by healthy people. But for diabetics it seems to increase insulin sensitivity and reduce the symptoms of nerve damage. Research is still ongoing and the doses for long-term use have not yet been determined.

Diabetics and supplements

When researching supplements on the internet I discovered lots of spurious claims that certain supplements can cure or prevent diseases, or provide you with energy. At the same time, I did discover some reliable sites that contain research-tested information. These are mainly connected to reputable universities, medical schools and teaching hospitals.

Most of the trustworthy websites state that eating a balance diet is the best way for a healthy person to get all the nutrients he or she needs. But, as you are diabetic, you are not healthy.

If you follow my diet for beating diabetes, you will be avoiding a major food group (dairy products), as well as cancelling eggs, and will be reducing your intake of meats and fish to an extremely-lean minimum.

Because you will be omitting a major good group from your diet you will probably be lacking certain micro-nutrients and therefore will need dietary supplements.

So what dietary supplements should you take?

Choosing your supplements

If you are trying to control your diabetes you are probably also trying to control high blood pressure and cholesterol levels. But the results of research into the efficacy of supplements in ameliorating these three conditions are clouded in uncertainty.

This is because it is difficult to control dietary factors in long-term research. In addition, a researcher can never be sure whether a deficiency in a micro-nutrient is a cause of, or is caused by, a particular disease.

Most medical scientists consider that taking one multivitamin a day is adequate. However, in order to ensure that you get adequate amounts of vitamins B12 and D, the American Medical Association recommends two-a-day ... besides one multi-vitamin, I take a separate supplement of vitamin B12 and a calcium tablet which includes vitamin D.

My research suggests that some medicines change the way the body uses nutrients. Interactions between any medicines you are taking and the nutrients in your food can sometimes cause a deficiency in a vitamin or mineral. For example, taking lots of aspirin can increase your need for iron. However, this whole area is fraught with unknown factors and gaps in knowledge.

You need to choose a supplement that combines a variety of vitamins and minerals in amounts that a right for you. The trick is to read the labels of several products before choosing. Note in particular the following which I turned up using internet research:

(1) **Iron** ... avoid this mineral. Most people have enough stored iron and do not need more unless they have a history of anaemia (in which case their doctor will advise them).

(2) **Vitamin A** ... maintains healthy skin and eyes. Get it as beta-carotene rather than preformed vitamin A (which can be toxic in large doses).

(3) **Vitamin C** ... assists in a variety of functions, including the protection of eyes and the absorption of iron. It is said to have anti-cancer properties. It seems to raise HDL (good) cholesterol levels while, along with beta-carotene and vitamin E, reducing the damaging effects of cholesterol in the blood.

(4) **Vitamin B12** ... is essential for healthy blood cells and the maintenance of normal nerve function. I can personally attest to its efficacy in reducing the effects of diabetic neuropathy. I try to take at least 5mcg a day which, as any excess is excreted in the urine, is not dangerous.

(5) **Vitamin D** ... helps you to absorb calcium and phosphorus (among other functions). You get it from the action of sunlight on your skin and from fish oils, egg yolks and liver. However, if you are following my diet to beat diabetes, these foods are off-limits and you should take a supplement, the recommended amount being 400 IU (international units) per day ... check the multi-vitamin you take and

if it does not give you 400 IU of vitamin D, take the vitamin as a separate supplement.

(6) **Vitamin B3 (niacin)** ... is used to lower LDL (bad) cholesterol and triglyceride (fat) levels. However it can raise blood glucose levels and clash with cholesterol-lowering medications, so you should not take high doses of niacin without your doctor's supervision.

(7) **Potassium** ... may cause a slight drop in blood pressure according to inconclusive evidence. At least 4.7gm per day is recommended. I eat a banana every morning to ensure that I get enough.

(8) **Selenium** ... may, in combination with vitamin E and beta-carotene, help lower LDL (bad) cholesterol. But be cautious about including it in your multivitamin as it can have a negative effect on cholesterol reducing drugs such as statins.

(9) **Zinc** ... is said to lower HDL (good) cholesterol and to raise LDL (bad) cholesterol, so it should be treated with caution.

(10) **Calcium** ... is usually included in a multi-vitamin supplement. However, you may need to take an extra calcium supplement as most combined supplements do not contain enough calcium to meet the recommended dietary intake for that mineral.

However, when you buy calcium as a separate supplement, make sure it includes vitamin D. A reputable manufacturer will ensure that the amount of vitamin D supplied in each tablet matches the amount of calcium.

Discussing the supplements you intend to take with your medical advisor first would be an ultra-smart idea because (a) you may need a particular supplement depending on your health, or (b) you may need to avoid certain supplements because they interfere with some medication you are taking.

Here's what I take each morning with my breakfast:

(1) Multivitamin

(2) B12 (4mcg) in a separate tablet
(3) Calcium (400mg) plus vitamin D (2.5mcg) together in a separate tablet
(4) High-strength cod-liver oil capsule with vitamins D and E, in a separate capsule
(5) Cinnamon ... one large teaspoon sprinkled on my porridge (oatmeal) or other cereal

The supplements I take are what I feel I need to maintain a full properly balanced diet. Each person however is different and has differing nutritional needs.

You need to tailor the supplements you take to your own actual nutritional needs through discussions with your medical advisor.

18 - Water

I used to despise water ... and seldom drank it unless there was
nothing else ... until I realised that it can play a crucial part in
beating diabetes by, among other things, helping you to move dietary
fibre through your system.

Water is, in fact, the second most vital substance (after air) for
animals. Indeed, it is essential for all organisms. And in human
beings, about 70% of the body by mass (excluding fat) is composed
of water. Even brain tissue, I have discovered, is 85% water.

Functions of water

Water has a variety of vital functions.

It is vital for the chemical reactions that take place during
metabolism (the changes that take place when various processes,
such as converting food to energy or getting rid of waste, are taking
place), and it carries nutrients and oxygen to the cells through the
blood.

Its role in metabolism means that water is a key factor in weight
loss. If you are trying to beat your diabetes you will probably need to
lose weight, but if you don't drink enough water, your body won't be
able to metabolize fat adequately.

Water also gets rid of wastes through urination, bowel
movements and perspiration. Indeed without it, we'd be poisoned to
death by our own waste. When the kidneys remove uric acid and
urea, these must be dissolved in water. If there isn't enough water,
wastes are not removed fully and you are likely to experience a
build-up of kidney stones.

Water performs a host of other functions. For example, it keeps
you cool through perspiration, and lubricates and cushions your
joints. It also protects your spinal cord and other sensitive tissues.
You even need water to breathe ... to take in oxygen and excrete
carbon dioxide your lungs need to be moist.

Daily requirements for water

Water is excreted from the body in many ways, in your urine and
faeces, by sweating, and as vapour when you exhale. It is possible to

lose half-a-litre (a pint) or so a day just by breathing and this loss of fluids has to be replaced.

On average, about 80% of our daily water requirement for water is satisfied by the beverages we drink, and the remaining 20% comes from food. The water content of food varies depending on what is being eaten. Obviously fruit and vegetables contain more than cereals. I was surprised to learn that some foods (such as celery, tomatoes, oranges and melons) are in fact 85% to 95% water.

The big question, of course, is how much water you should drink every day. Using internet research I could not get a plain simple answer to this question. There is no real consensus among doctors and medical scientists.

I've often heard it suggested that the minimum water consumption needed to maintain proper hydration is six to eight glasses a day. However, I was unable to trace this recommendation to a credible source on the internet.

But I did find that overviews of the scientific literature carried out in 2002 and 2008 were also not able to find any reasons for the eight-glasses-a-day recommendation. And recent surveys of recommendations on fluid intake show wide variations in the volumes of water recommended for good health.

The current guidelines issued by the European Food Safety Authority (EFSA) recommend total water intakes of 2.0 litres a day for adult women and 2.5 l/d for adult men. These values include water from drinking water, other beverages, and from food. However, in the US, the reference daily intake (RDI) for water is 3.7 litres per day for males and 2.7 l/d for females, both over 18, obtained from all beverages and food.

I don't know why there are such wide discrepancies in these recommendations. In addition, I don't think that these recommendations are of much practical value ... it's easy enough to figure out how much fluid (water, coffee, tea, soft drinks, etc) you drink every day ... but how do you know how much water there is in the food you eat?

Common sense suggests that the amount of water needed will vary from person to person, and that it will depend on the state of a person's health, the amount of physical exercise they undertake, and on the temperature and humidity where they live and work. I feel that your thirst is a better guide as to how much water you require rather than any specific quantity.

Personally I drink about two litres (67 oz) of plain water a day. This is on top of another 2 litres or so in the form of coffee and tea. The diet I follow to beat my diabetes is a high roughage one and much of the fibre I eat is probably water-soluble.

Thus I feel that I need plenty of water in order to make the best use of this dietary fibre so that it can do its job of getting food and waste through my system and back out into the void. Four litres a day on top of what's in my food seems to work.

However, if you have a health problem, such as kidney disease, you may need to restrict your fluid intake. My best advice is that you discuss the matter thoroughly with your doctor and follow his or her advice.

Section Three: What Foods

I was determined to share my positive approach and not let diabetes stand in the way of enjoying my life ... Paula Deen

The purpose of this section is to help you decide what particular foods you should or should not eat.

Warning: all the information in this section was obtained through research on the internet. Thus, it may not be wholly accurate. Nevertheless, this background knowledge did help me to refine my diet so that I can go on beating my diabetes.

19 – Food in Three Varieties

So there you have it. To beat your diabetes all you need to do is to eat food that is ... natural ... low in sugar ... low in fat ... low in salt ... high in fibre ... and has low GI values. Your diet should consist mostly of plants. You should also drink lots of water.

If you follow this diet, you have a better than a 90% chance of controlling your disease successfully and avoiding the horrendous consequences of type 2 diabetes.

But what kinds of foods should you eat? What kinds should you avoid?

In my research on the internet, I discovered that there are various ways in which foods can be classified, depending on the criteria (such as nutritional values) chosen.

After considering these, I concluded that, in order to help me beat my diabetes, the most useful way to classify foods is as ... grains ... legumes ... vegetables ... fruits ... unprocessed meats ... processed meats ... eggs, and ... dairy products.

I also group these eight types of food into three different categories: (a) eat-all-you-want foods, (b) eat-only-a-little foods, and (c) don't-eat-at-all foods. These three very simple groups help me to make sense of the almost infinite variety of food available these days.

The (a) eat-all-you-want foods are types that fulfil the specific criteria of my diet ... that a food should be natural, low in sugar, low in fat, low in salt, high in fibre, and have a low GI value.

The other two categories fail to meet this standard either partly or wholly.

It seems reasonable to assume that grains, legumes, vegetables and fruits all fall into the (a) eat-all-you-want category. Unfortunately this is not so. You can eat all you want of whole-grain bread, for example, but white bread made from refined flour is in the (c) don't-eat-at-all category.

I feel it is important to remember that I am not eating my special diet just to beat my diabetes. I also what a diet that will help me control my cholesterol and blood pressure levels ... and, if possible, one that will also help to defend me against other diseases, such as cancers.

Rather than list all the foods you can eat (a vast range) it is easier to list all the foods you cannot eat, the no-noes or don't-eat-at-all category. To beat your diabetes, you need to avoid:

- the fat of meat, poultry, and fish
- eggs (whites and yolks)
- all dairy products (even if fat-free) such as milk, yogurt, cheese, ice cream, cream, sour cream, butter, etc
- added oils, eg, margarine, salad dressings, mayonnaise, cooking oils, etc
- fried foods, eg, potato chips, chips, French fries, onion rings, doughnuts, etc
- avocados, olives, and peanut butter
- refined foods
- foods with high GI (glycemic index) values, eg, white bread and white potatoes

20 - Grains

Grains, small hard seeds, are a fundamental part of the diet in all cultures. They can be eaten in three broad ways ... as porridges ... as baked products, and ... as berries in salads or side-dishes.

Grains make for healthy eating. They contain very little vegetable fat, no animal fat and no cholesterol.

But not all grains are equally healthful and, to beat your diabetes, you need to know what grains or grain products you can eat, ie you need some insight into what grains contain and how they are processed.

What's in a grain?
I researched this question on the internet and here's what I found out. All grains consist of three main parts ... the endosperm ... germ, and ... bran.

Endosperm is the main tissue inside the seeds. It provides nutrition in the form of starch, protein and oils.

The *germ* is the embryo, the reproductive part that germinates and grows into a plant. It is surrounded by the endosperm. The germ contains several essential nutrients. Wheat germ, for example, is a concentrated source of vitamin E, folate, phosphorus, thiamine, zinc and magnesium, essential fatty acids and fatty alcohols.

Bran is the hard outer layer of grain. It is rich in dietary fibre and essential fatty acids and contains starch (the most common carbohydrate in our diets), protein, vitamins and minerals.

When cereal grains are harvested they also have an outer *husk*. This tough protective coating needs to be removed by threshing (beating them) and winnowing (blowing away the chaff, broken off bits of husk) before you can eat the grains.

Groats are the grains after threshing. Though the husk has gone groats still include the bran and the germ. Groats are nutritious but hard to chew so they have to be prepared by soaking and cooking.

Whole grains v refined grains
There are two types of grains we can eat: whole grains and refined grains.

Whole grains are cereal grains in their natural state, ie, as well as the endosperm, they also contain the bran and germ. They fall into the eat-all-you-want category of foods, as a general rule.

Refined grains are groats from which the bran and germ have been removed by grinding and sifting. Refining causes the grains to lose some of their nutritional value.

Sometimes thiamine, riboflavin, niacin, and iron may be added back. But, as the added nutrients represent a small fraction of the nutrients removed, refined grains are nutritionally much inferior to whole grains.

Removing the fibre and grinding the grains finely also increases the glycemic index value, ie glucose from refined grains is digested quicker by the body than glucose from whole grains, which is not what you want as a diabetic.

Though whole grains are loaded with carbohydrates, in countries where whole-grains are staples, diabetes is much less common than in North America and Europe ... mainly due to the high fibre content in the bran of the whole grains, which slows the release of glucose.

Going for whole-grains

Whole grains are great for our health in many other ways, thanks to their high levels of vitamins and minerals. Most whole grains, including brown rice and oats, are particularly rich in B vitamins.

Whole grains also have plenty of protein, up to 10 grams in a 1/2-cup serving. One of these proteins is gluten. Gluten makes dough elastic, which helps it to rise and keep its shape. It constitutes about 80% of the protein in wheat seed, which is one reason why wheat is popular for bread-making. It is also found in barley and rye.

For these reasons I stick to whole-grains. Instead of white bread, I eat whole-grain bread. Instead of white rice I eat brown rice. I always start the day with a bowl of porridge (oatmeal) fortified with bran, wheat-germ, cinnamon, a banana and half a mug of mixed berries.

However, I've learned that you have to be careful when shopping ... not all breads and crackers labelled as 'whole grain' are the real deal. You have to read the labels carefully. If the product is high in fat, you can be fairly sure it is not whole-grain. And if it's high in fat, you should not eat it anyway.

Whole grains come in many forms ... brown rice, wheat, oats, millet, barley, and so on. These grains are processed into a variety of products ... pasta, couscous, bulgur wheat, whole-grain breads, pumpernickel or rye bread, porridge (oatmeal) bran, almost ad infinitum.

Most, but not all, are healthful. Here's what I found on the internet.

Wheat

Wheat is the most important staple food for humans. Indeed it is our leading source of vegetable protein, having a higher protein content than either maize (corn) or rice.

Wheat grain is used to make bread, biscuits (cookies), crackers, cakes, muffins, doughnuts, porridge (oatmeal), breakfast cereals, pastry, pasta, noodles, and couscous. It is also fermented to make beer and other alcoholic drinks, and can be used as biofuel.

As a food, wheat is highly nutritious but its nutritional content differs between varieties ... of which the two most important are common (or bread) wheat and durum (or hard) wheat.

Proteins (including gluten) can range from 10% in soft wheats (with high starch contents) to over 15% in hard wheats. The amount of fat varies but is nearly always below 2%, while up to 12.5% or 1/8th can consist of fibre. Carbohydrate (mainly starch) makes up about 70% of a wheat grain.

Wheat also contains significant amounts of iron, and is also rich in the B vitamins and dietary minerals. Unfortunately these, along with wheat's fibre, tend to disappear during processing, ie, the milling (grinding) that separates the bran and germ from the endosperm to produce refined flour.

Brown rice

To produce brown rice from paddy (freshly harvested rice) only the husk (outermost layer of the grain) is removed. When the next layers, the bran and the germ, are removed, leaving mostly the starchy endosperm, the result is white rice.

The number of calories and carbohydrates in brown and white rice are similar. Their nutritional contents, however, are very different. Several vitamins and minerals, such as some B vitamins, iron and magnesium, are lost when the bran and germ are removed. Other losses include the oil in the bran (which may help lower LDL cholesterol), fatty acids and fibre.

The only draw-back I can see to brown rice is that it goes rancid more quickly because the germ, which is removed to make white rice, contains fats that can spoil.

Oats & Oatmeal

Oats are a super-nutritious grain. They are full of high quality protein ... from 12 to 24% ... the highest among all cereals. Oat protein is nearly the equivalent in quality to the protein in soy, meat, milk and egg, according to the WHO.

Whole oats are excellent sources of thiamine and iron. They are the only source of avenanthramides, antioxidant compounds believed to help protect the circulatory system from arteriosclerosis.

Oats are rich in fibre. While rice and wheat contain lots of insoluble fibre, the fibre in oats is soluble. Indeed, oats contain more soluble fibre (10% or more) than any other grain, which means they have a lower GI, and greater fill-you-up power. With oats you feel full for longer.

Beta-glucan, a type of soluble fibre found in oats (and in barley), has been proved to lower blood cholesterol levels. Beta-glucan may also help type 2 diabetics bring their blood-glucose levels under control and may stimulate the immune system to fight off bacterial infections.

Rolled oats are oat groats that have been flattened into flakes under heavy rollers and then steamed and lightly toasted. *Thick-rolled oats* are whole flakes and *thin-rolled oats* are small fragmented flakes. *Steel-cut oats* are groats that have been chopped into smaller pieces yet still retain bits of the bran layer. All types are known as *oatmeal*.

Since the nutritious bran layer makes the grains tough to chew and also contains an enzyme that can cause the oats to go rancid, raw groats are often steam-treated to soften them in order to speed up cooking and to neutralise the enzymes for a longer shelf life.

Oatmeal is used to make porridge and baked goods, such as bread, cakes and biscuits (cookies), and as part of the mix in muesli and granola. Oats may be eaten raw, and some biscuits contain raw oats.

Oat flakes that are simply rolled whole oats without further processing can be cooked and eaten as 'old-fashioned' porridge or oatmeal. More fragmented and processed rolled oats absorb water much more easily and cook faster.

As it is less nutritious, you should avoid 'quick' or 'instant' oatmeal to which you just add boiling water to make your porridge. Choose oatmeal that you have to bring to the boil and simmer or cook in a micro-wave oven.

Rolled oats that are sold as oatmeal very often have had the bran removed, but it's difficult to tell this from the labelling. For this reason I always add pure oat bran to my porridge in the morning.

Barley

Barley is highly nutritious. While raw barley is 77.7% carbohydrates, less than 1% is sugar. Only 1.2% is fat, and nearly 10% is protein. Barley also contains eight essential amino acids. In addition, fibre makes up more than 15% of raw barley, which also contains a string of B vitamins and minerals such as calcium, magnesium, phosphorus, iron, and potassium.

It is definitely worth fitting barley into your diet.

Much of the fibre in barley is soluble and, like oats, includes beta-glucan which, as mentioned above, lowers cholesterol, and may help control glucose levels and stimulate the immune system.

Barley has a low GI value. According to a recent study I found, eating whole-grain barley can reduce blood glucose response to a meal for up to 10 hours after consumption compared to white or even whole-grain wheat which has a similar glycemic index value. This is attributed to the fermentation of indigestible carbohydrates in the colon.

The best thing of all about barley is that it tastes pretty good and has a great texture. You'll find it in breakfast cereals and in some types of bread. It's great in porridges, gruels, soups and stews, and you can use it as a side-dish of grain. Or you can mix it with rice and cook them both together.

When buying barley, however, you need to read the information on the package carefully. *Hulled barley* (aka *pot barley* or *scotch barley*) is a whole grain which still has its bran and germ as only the outer hull has been removed, which makes it a healthy food.

Pearl or *pearled barley* is hulled barley from which the bran has been removed by steaming. Pearl barley may also be polished in a process known as pearling (hence the name).

Both hulled and pearl barley are used in a variety of barley products, including barley flour, barley flakes or meal (similar to oatmeal) and grits. Read the labels.

Malts

Malts are germinated cereal grains that have been dried by 'malting'. The grains are soaked in water to make them germinate. Germination is then halted by drying the grains with hot air.

Malting develops the enzymes required to modify the grain's starches into sugars. It also develops other enzymes that which break down the proteins into forms that can be used by yeast.

Malted grain is used to make beer, whisky, malted shakes, malt vinegar, chocolate confections such as Maltesers and Whoppers, flavoured drinks (eg, Horlicks, Ovaltine and Milo), and baked goods such as malt loaf.

All types of cereals can be malted, but barley is the most common. A high-protein form of malted barley is often used in blended flours in the manufacture of yeast breads and other baked goods.

As a diabetic you will naturally avoid the Maltesers and similar chocolates, as well as the flavoured drinks as these invariably include milk and other dairy products.

Indeed most malted products are out of bounds but you should be able to eat malt loaf provided it has not been doused with sugar.

Rye

Rye is my favourite grain for reasons of taste and health. It is closely related to barley and wheat and is used for flour, rye bread and crisp bread, and can also be eaten whole, either as boiled rye berries, or by being rolled, similar to rolled oats.

You can buy rye as a whole grain, cracked grains, flour or flakes. The flour has less gluten than wheat and very little fat. Rye contains a higher proportion of soluble fibre. Foods made from rye, such as pumpernickel bread, have a full, hearty taste.

Rye is a great source of fibre containing non-cellulose polysaccharides, which have very high water-binding capacity. These quickly give a feeling of satiety. Rye has plenty of magnesium, which acts as a co-factor for enzymes involved in the body's use of glucose and the secretion of insulin. Research suggests that regular consumption lowers the risk of type 2 diabetes substantially for healthy people.

Rye bread may also be a better choice than wheat bread for persons with diabetes. According to Finnish researchers, insulin responses are significantly lower after eating rye bread compared to wheat bread. The researchers attribute this to the fibre content of rye and to the fact that the starch granules in rye bread form a less porous matrix than in wheat bread, so that larger particles of bread are swallowed which, in turn, slows the rate at which the starch can be digested into sugar.

Since its gluten is less elastic than that of wheat and it holds less gas during leavening, breads made with rye are more compact and dense, which gives them their 'heaviness'. As it is difficult to separate the germ and bran from the endosperm of rye, rye flour usually retains a greater quantity of nutrients compared to wheat flour, making rye a super-healthy choice.

German pumpernickel is made from crushed or ground whole rye grains. Made only with rye flour, it is heavy and chewy. I love it but many people don't, at least not the pure rye version. So, rye and wheat flours may be mixed to make bread which has a lighter texture than pumpernickel.

Rye bread recipes typically include ground spices such as fennel, coriander, aniseed, cardamom, or citrus peel. Caraway seeds are also added quite often.

Pure-rye breads can keep for a long times, for months rather than days, and are popular for this reason. Because they are so dense, pure-rye breads are sold already cut into very thin slices.

Millets

Millets are a group of cereal grasses with smaller seeds than other grains. There are several types ... pearl millet ... finger millet ... small millet ... barnyard millet.

The protein content of millets is about 11%, similar to wheat and maize. However, millets do not contain any gluten, so they can only be used for flat breads or porridges. Roti, the well known flat-bread of India, is made from millet.

The fat content of millets varies ... pearl and little millet are the highest in fat while finger millet contains less fat than the other types. Millets are full of carbohydrates in the form of starch.

The bran layers of millets are good sources of B-complex vitamins. Millets are rich in dietary minerals ... iron, calcium, phosphorus, potassium, magnesium, and zinc. They are also high in fibre.

But their nutrients are difficult to digest which severely limits their nutritional value. Finger millet, for example, has the highest calcium content of all the food grains, but it is not easily assimilated. For this reason, I was surprised to notice that many health-food shops promote millet as a sort of wondrous food with all sorts of health benefits.

Semolina

Semolina is the coarse middlings of durum wheat.

Coarse middlings are the particles of bran, wheat germ and other residues left after wheat (or rice and corn) is milled into flour.

Wheat is milled into flour using grooved steel rollers, which are adjusted so that the space between them is slightly narrower than the width of the wheat kernels. When the wheat is fed into the mill, the rollers flake off the bran and germ and break the endosperm into coarse pieces. The endosperm is separated out by sifting and the remainder (mainly the bran and the germ) is semolina.

Ground into flour, semolina is an intermediate product in the making of couscous, pasta etc. When boiled it turns into a mushy porridge and can be eaten as either a savoury or sweetened dish.

The bran and germ contained in all forms of semolina makes then very nutritious.

The downer for diabetics is the ingredients, sugar for example, that manufacturers insist on adding to products such as semolina pudding. In particular, you need to be wary of the Middle Eastern deserts made from semolina, such as helwa.

Bulgur wheat

Bulgur is a quick-cooking form of whole wheat that has been parboiled (partially pre-cooked) and dried. It is usually made from durum wheat, though in the USA common wheat is used. It is not the same as *cracked wheat*, which is crushed wheat grain that has not been parboiled.

Bulgur may be sold as whole kernels but it is usually ground into particles which are sifted and sold in various sizes. Because only a small amount of bran is removed during processing, it is considered a whole grain. It has a pleasant, nutty flavour, and can be stored for long periods.

Best of all, bulgur is highly nutritious. A 100gm contains nearly 16g of carbohydrates (of which less than half a gram are sugars), 12.29g of protein, and only 1.33g of fat. Just 3.5% of the energy in bulgur comes from fat.

Bulgur is also high in dietary fibre (more than 18%) and rich in B vitamins, iron, phosphorus and manganese.

This grain has more nutritional impact than rice or couscous.

Bulgur also requires very little cooking. It was the first instant food, invented by the ancient Bulgarians (about whom nothing else is known) nearly 8,000 years ago.

It can be mixed with other ingredients without being cooked. It can be used in pilaffs (rice cooked with meat or vegetables), casseroles, soups, baked goods, or as stuffing. It can be used to add whole-grains in bread. It is often served as a side dish, like rice, couscous or pasta, or as a meat substitute in vegetarian dishes. It is used in common Middle Eastern dishes such as tabbouleh salad and kibbeh.

Bulgur's high nutritional value and versatility makes it an ideal grain for beating your diabetes.

Couscous

Couscous is made from semolina, which is sprinkled with water, rolled into pellets and dried.

It is one of the healthiest grain-based products there is ... each 100g contains 12.76g of protein, 77.43g of carbohydrates (of which only 1g is sugar), only 0.64g of fat, and 5g of dietary fibre.

It also has a fairly full range of minerals, including sodium, potassium, magnesium, phosphorus, zinc, calcium, iron, copper, and manganese. Though couscous does not contain any vitamin C, it has plenty of B vitamins, as well as vitamins A and D.

Couscous is nutritionally superior to pasta as it contains twice as much riboflavin, niacin, vitamin B6, and folate and four times as much thiamine and pantothenic acid. In addition, its glycemic load per gram is 25% below that of pasta. Moreover, the fat-to-calorie ratio of couscous is 1%, compared to 3% for white rice, 5% for pasta, and 11.3% for rice pilaf.

There are hundreds of ways to eat couscous. In North Africa it is served under a stew of vegetables, meat or fish, or as a sweet dessert of steamed couscous (into which dates, almonds, raisins, cinnamon and so on have been mixed). In South America, you can try it as a steamed cake under either savoury or sweet toppings. In Mexico, it is added to tacos and burritos.

Or, you can use it as a substitute for potatoes, rice or pasta on the traditional Western dinner plate ... which is what I do.

Noodles

Noodles are made from unleavened dough which is rolled flat and cut into shapes ... thin strips, wavy strips, tubes, strings, shells, etc.

They can be made from many grains and legumes, including wheat, rice, buckwheat, acorns, and mung beans. Some noodles include egg (eg, pasta).

Instant noodles are made by flash-frying fresh noodles which are then dried out to give them a long shelf life.

Noodles are very versatile. They can be boiled in water then drained and served under a sauce, cooked in a broth with meat, fish or vegetables, stir-fried with meat, seafood, vegetables and dairy products, or added to casseroles. They can also be served cold in salads.

The nutritional value of noodles will depend on what they are made from and how they are made, and will vary enormously from type to type.

Typical values for 100g of cooked noodles are about 14 grams of protein, 71 grams of carbohydrates, 4 grams of fat (relatively high), and 3g of dietary fibre. They have a medium GI value. Noodles usually also contain some Vitamin A, Vitamin B3 and folate, as well as phosphorus, a little iron, potassium, magnesium and sodium.

Though nutritional values vary widely from one type of noodle to another, noodles may be a useful alternative to other starchy carbohydrates. To judge whether they will help you beat your diabetes, you need to read the product labels. Look out for wholegrain varieties and watch for excessive fat.

Pasta

Pasta is a type of noodle. It can be fresh or dried, though dried is the most common type. Both types come in an amazing number of shapes ... long strings, short strings, tubes, flat tapes and sheets, and miniature alphabets, among many others. The shapes can also be filled or stuffed.

Pasta is simple but very versatile. It can be served as the bed for a nutritious sauce (eg, spaghetti Bolognese). It can be added to a soup to create a heavy broth or incorporated into a dish that is baked (eg, lasagne). Cold pasta also goes well in a salad of mixed vegetables.

Pasta is usually made from wheat flour or semolina, though other grains such as barley, buckwheat, rye, rice and maize, as well as chestnut or chickpea flour, can be used. It is nearly always made from unleavened dough, though there are at least nine pastas made from yeast-raised doughs.

To make pasta, the semolina or flour is mixed with water and formed into sheets or various shapes. Instead of water, chicken eggs, duck eggs, milk or cream, may be used. The basic flour-liquid mixture can be augmented with vegetables purees such as spinach or tomato, mushrooms, cheeses, herbs, spices and other seasonings, as a quick glance through the shelves in any supermarket will confirm.

Dried pasta has a long shelf life. Eggs are usually added to the semolina flour for flavour and richness after which the pasta is dried for several days to get rid of all the moisture. Dried pasta usually doubles in size during cooking.

On the face of it, pasta is a healthful food. A 100g of pasta delivers 350 calories, 11 to 12g of protein, approximately 79g of carbohydrates (of which soluble sugars are only just over 4g) but only about 1g or so of fat. A 100g of pasta also has 2.7g of fibre (of which 1.15g or 43% is soluble).

But pasta contains few vitamins and minerals, except potassium, though some pasta is enriched with iron and B vitamins. However pasta is usually combined with nutritious foods, such as beans, vegetables, fish, tomato sauces and lean ground beef, so meals based on pasta are usually healthful.

Pasta has a low glycemic index, provided it is unleavened and not overcooked. Unleavened pasta has no air-pockets into which your digestive juices can enter and break the molecules of semolina down quickly into glucose.

But pasta must be cooked al-dente (still chewy). If you overcook it, the pasta will expand and enable rapid digestion. The longer you cook pasta, the higher its GI value.

For this reason I am a bit chary of pasta. I have discovered that if pasta is more than barely cooked, or I eat more than just a little, my blood glucose will be higher than usual two hours after my meal.

Summary

To beat your diabetes you need to choose wholemeal rather than refined grains and breads, and go for brown rice rather than white rice.

The best grains for beating diabetes are bulgur, couscous, rye and barley, which can be added to other dishes or used as a side-dish in a main course. But eat hulled barley and avoid pearl or pearled barley.

Make your morning porridge (oatmeal) from rolled oats and add pure oat-bran to porridge. Avoid 'quick' or 'instant' porridge.

Eat rye berries and rye bread. Avoid all malts or malted grains except for sugar-free malt loaf.

Only eat a little millet.

Go for semolina products provided (and only provided) they are sugar-free.

Be careful with noodles, and only eat pasta if it is cooked al-dente.

21 - Grain Products

Grain products range from breakfast food through the carbohydrates we eat for dinner to a vast range of baked products. As a general rule, you can eat all you want (within reason) of foods based on whole grains but should be very cautious of foods made using refined grains. But watch out for added sugar.

Breakfast cereals

Breakfast cereals are grain-based foods such as porridge (oatmeal), bran, and cold cereals. Many come in ready-to-eat form. They can be served as warm or cold cereals.

Porridge (oatmeal) ... provided it is made using whole-rolled oats or other wholemeal grains, there is no better way for a diabetic to start the day. But you can eat porridges at other times during the day.

In China, rice congee (which may have cornmeal or millet added) is a popular porridge. Porridge for children is made in Greece by boiling cornmeal and milk. Kasha, porridge of buckwheat or other grains, is eaten in Russia, Poland and Croatia. Pap, a South African porridge, is made from maize and eaten throughout the day.

Ready-to-eat cereals include both warm and cold breakfast cereals.

Ready-to-cook porridge oats have been around since 1877. The problem with ready-to-cook porridges (for diabetics) is that sweeteners, such as brown sugar, honey or maple syrup are often added during manufacturing.

Corn flakes are a popular ready-to-eat cold cereal and were once considered a health food.

Muesli, a mixture of uncooked rolled oats, fruit and nuts, was developed around 1900 by a Swiss doctor. Instead of buying packaged versions, which often have sugar added, you can easily make up your own. But you need to leave out the nuts (due to their fat) as well as the sugar.

In the 20th century, new ready-to-eat cold breakfast cereals were developed to target children. Marketing ploys included the creation and introduction of a range of mascots, such as the Rice Krispies elves and other characters like Tony the Tiger.

The problem was that many of the healthy aspects of breakfast cereals were altered in order to appeal to the palates of children. Sugar was added to improve flavour, while fibre was removed to (supposedly) make digestion and the absorption of nutrients easier.

Hard to believe but at one time, Kellogg's Sugar Smacks contained 56% sugar by weight!

Baked products

In baking, food is cooked in an oven using dry heat acting by convection (rather than thermal radiation as in grilling). Roasting is similar to baking except that it involves higher temperatures and shorter cooking times.

Baking does not require fat during cooking, unlike frying, which should make food prepared in this way attractive to type 2 diabetics ... the problem lies in the ingredients in baked products.

There are three general categories of baked grain products ... breads ... pastries and ... cakes.

Breads

Bread is made with dough, a paste of flour and water. This is usually leavened, allowed to rise, and then baked in an oven. Breads may contain additional ingredients, such as salt or butter, to improve taste.

Flour ... is grain that has been ground into a powder. It is usually made from common wheat because this flour has high levels of gluten, which gives the dough sponginess and elasticity.

But bread is also made from other species of wheat (eg, durum and spelt) and other grains such as rye, barley, corn (maize) and oats. The non-wheat grains are usually combined with wheat flour.

The quality of the bread depends largely on the protein content of the flour. The best breads use flour with 12–14% protein rather than all-purpose wheat flour which only contains 9–12% protein.

Liquids ... are used to turn the flour into dough. Water is the most usual but other liquids, such as diary products, beer or fruit juices, can be used. As well as the water they contain, these liquids contribute fats, leavening components and/or sweeteners to the bread.

Leavening ... is the adding of gas to the dough before or during cooking to make it rise (swell up) so that the bread is lighter and easier to chew. There are several ways this can be done (see below).

Improvers ... are additives used to quicken the rising time, increase volume and enhance texture. They can include ascorbic acid and ammonium chloride.

Salt is one of the most common improvers. It enhances the flavour and affects the crumb (or inside of the bread) by strengthening the gluten.

Fats ... have a role in bread-making. They include butter, vegetable oils, lard or the fat contained in eggs. These shortenings, as they are known, are solids at room temperature and help to keep the structure together by affecting the development of the gluten.

A fat content of about 3% by weight is considered best to enhance leavening. Fats also help tenderise bread and preserve its freshness.

Cooking ... is usually by baking in an oven. But bread can be made by frying in oil (eg, Indian puri), baking on a dry (unoiled) frying pan (eg, Mexican tortillas) and by steaming (eg, Chinese mantou).

Leavening

Leavening is a way of making grain products lighter and thus easier to digest by creating bubbles within the dough.

When flour and water are combined to make dough, the starch in the flour mixes with the water to form a matrix. When this mixture is leavened, ie gas is added, the dough 'rises'. Then, when it sets, the bubbles remain trapped in the dough.

Dough can be leavened using biological agents, chemical agents or mechanical means. Most types of bread are leavened using biological agents containing micro-organisms that release carbon dioxide as part of their life-cycle and are either yeasts or sourdough starters.

Yeast ... ferments some of the carbohydrates in the flour and produces carbon dioxide, which makes the dough rise.

Commercially-produced baker's yeast is used by most bakeries in the West because it is quick and reliable.

This kind of leavening requires proofing, ie a resting time to allow the yeast to reproduce and consume carbohydrates. Yeast leavened breads have a distinctive flavour.

Sourdough starter ... is a paste of flour and water containing yeast and lactobacilli which has been obtained from a previous batch of dough.

Each time they bake bread, bakers who use this technique reserve a lump of dough as a starter for the next batch. Starters can be maintained by just adding flour and water, and some are several generations old.

A sourdough starter works in the same way as yeast, by creating bubbles, and also requires proofing time. The bacteria in sourdough give it a sour, tangy taste. Its disadvantage is the lengthy time it takes the dough to rise compared to baker's yeast.

Sourdough is used for rye-based breads where yeast is not really effective in leavening the dough.

Chemical leaveners ... are chemical mixtures that release carbon dioxide or other gases when they react to moisture and heat.

There are two methods of chemical leavening. The first uses baking powder (or self-raising flour that contains baking powder), while the second way is to add buttermilk (which is acidic) and baking soda to the dough... the reaction of the acid and the soda makes the gas.

Chemical leaveners not need a long fermentation period, and are used for 'quick breads' such as Irish soda bread, banana bread, pancakes, carrot cake and muffins.

Mechanical means ... can be used to introduce bubbles into a mixture.

In *creaming*, sugar crystals and butter (solid fat) are beaten together in a mixer. The crystals cut through the structure of the fat which integrates tiny bubbles into the mixture. Creamed mixtures are used for biscuits (cookies).

In *whisking*, foams of certain liquids (notably cream or egg whites) are created. Whisking is used in the making of sponge cakes in which the egg protein matrix made by whisking provides almost all the structure of the finished cake.

The **Chorleywood Bread Process** ... a mix of biological and mechanical leavening, is used to make about 80% of British bread because it is considered the best way to deal with the soft wheat grown in Britain.

Critics say it is less nutritious than bread made using traditional leavening agents.

The big question for diabetics, of course, is whether the rising method has any effect on the glycemic index (GI) of the bread. The intuitive answer is that it must worsen the GI because it introduces air into the matrix.

But according to recent research, this is not true. A study in New Zealand indicates that the leavening agents used in making bread do not have any impact on the GI of the bread.

Different kinds of breads

There are hundreds of different breads in the world. Here are some of the most common:

White bread ... is made from refined flour, ie grain from which the bran and germ have been removed so that it only contains the endosperm (central core of the grain)

Brown bread ... is white bread to which colouring (usually caramel based) has been added to make it brown; it may also have added bran (up to 10%)

Wholemeal bread ... is made from the whole of the wheat grain (endosperm, bran, and germ), ie from unrefined flour

Wheat germ bread ... has added wheat germ for flavouring

Whole-grain bread ... is white bread to which whole grains have been added to increase its fibre content; eg, '60% whole-grain bread'

Granary bread ... is made from flaked wheat grains and white or brown flour

Rye bread ... is made with rye grain; it has more fibre than most other breads, a darker colour and a stronger flavour

Crisp bread ... is a flat and dry type of bread or cracker, made mostly of rye flour

Matzo ... is unleavened bread

Flatbread ... is made from unleavened dough of flour, water and salt; a few are made with yeast

Roti ... is unleavened whole-wheat bread; chapatti is the large version of roti; naan is the leavened equivalent

Quick breads ... chemically leavened breads such as Irish soda bread

Pastry

The main difference between pastry and bread is that pastry contains more fat. It's the fat that gives pastry its texture. Pastry also has a greater range of ingredients ... flour ... sugar ... milk ... butter ... shortening (fat that is solid at room temperature) ... baking powder, and/or ... eggs.

These ingredients make pastries much less suitable for beating your diabetes compared to bread.

Pastry dough can be used as a base or cover for dishes such as tarts, quiches and pies. It may be shaped into cases for sweet or savoury mixtures. It can also be used to create a product on its own such as croissants and brioches.

There are several kinds of pastry in Western cuisine:

Short-crust pastry ... is a simple pastry made from flour, fat, butter, salt and water. First the flour and fat are mixed before water is added and the dough is rolled out. It's the most common pastry.

Sweet-crust pastry ... is similar to short-crust pastry except that it has been sweetened with sugar.

Puff pastry ... is a leavened pastry made from flour, butter, salt and water. Once mixed and allowed to rise, the dough is rolled out flat and spread with solid fat. It is folded and rolled out again several times and the fat is spread each time.

During baking, the air between the layers expands so that the dough puffs up and the pastry comes out of the oven light and flaky. Puff pastry is used for making turnovers, pies, sausage rolls, strudels etc.

Flaky pastry ... is similar to puff pastry except that it is unleavened. Like puff pastry it is repeatedly rolled out but, instead of the fat being spread across the layer, chunks of shortening are used to keep the rolled particles of dough separate from each other so that they turn into flakes when they are baked.

Flaky pastry is used to make pasties, turnovers, sausage rolls and plaits.

Phyllo (Filo) pastry ... consists of paper-thin sheets of unleavened flour dough used for making pastries in Middle Eastern and Balkan cuisine. The dough is made with flour, water, and a small amount of oil and raki (Turkish alcohol aperitif) or white vinegar; egg yolks are also used sometimes.

The dough is usually stacked in layers rather than being folded (as in puff pastry). A filling may be inserted between the layers or the layers of dough are ruffled up and wrapped around a (sweet or savoury) filling. It is often brushed with butter or egg yolk before baking.

Examples of phyllo pastries include baklava (filled with syrup and nuts) and tiropita (filled with cheese).

Choux pastry ... is made from a light dough containing only butter, water, flour and eggs. Its high moisture content creates steam during baking which puffs up the pastry.

It is used for making éclairs and profiteroles and similar concoctions which are usually filled with flavoured cream and topped with chocolate ... hardly a help in beating your diabetes.

Viennoiseries ... are made from a yeast-leavened dough similar to a bread dough or from puff pastry but with added ingredients such as eggs, butter, milk, cream and sugar which give them a rich sweet taste. Examples include croissant and brioche.

Western pastry is based on flour. However traditional pastry-making in Asia is based on rice or a mixture of rice and flour.

Old Chinese recipes use rice dough to enclose fruit, sweet bean paste or sesame-based fillings. Rice, flour and fruit are used in Korea and Japan to make pastry-based desserts.

Oriental pastries are generally less sweet than Western recipes and would probably be a better bet for beating your diabetes.

Cakes
Deciding whether a particular baked product should be classified as

bread, pastry or cake can be difficult. What we know as cakes are in fact highly-sweetened bread-like foods. A cake, in other words, is simply a sweet baked dessert.

Most cakes are made from flour, sugar, eggs and butter or oil, and may also require water or milk and a leavening agent such as yeast or baking powder. Nuts and fruit (pureed, dried or candied) are often added to the mix for flavour; viz, fruit cake.

Cakes can be divided into several broad categories based on their ingredients and how they are cooked:

Yeast cakes ... are made in a similar way to yeast breads. The difference is that they are doused in honey or some other sweetener.

Sponge cakes ... are not made with yeast and leavening is provided by air trapped in a protein matrix (usually of beaten eggs) along with a bit of baking powder. Gateaux are sponge cakes with lavish, highly decorated toppings.

Butter cakes ... get their leavening and moist texture from a combination of butter and eggs and a dash of baking powder. Prime examples are pound cake and devil's food cake.

Cheesecakes ... are not really cakes at all. In fact they are more like pastry tarts or cases with a filling based on cheese that has been sweetened with honey or another kind of syrup.

The flour used to make cakes is ground from soft, fine-textured, low-protein wheat, which gives a lighter, less dense texture than all-purpose flour.

Many cakes are filled with jam, preserved fruit, pastry cream or other dessert sauces. They may be enhanced with an outer cover of icing, frosting, and/or marzipan, and decorated with candied fruit, piped borders and sprinkles (hard coloured pieces of oiled sugar).

There are various kinds of icing. All are made with icing sugar, ie powdered or finely ground sugar.

Butter cream ... is an icing made by creaming a mixture of butter and icing sugar.

It is used to cover sponge cakes and butter cakes.

Royal icing ... is a hard white icing made from beaten egg whites and icing sugar.

It is used on fruit cakes such as Christmas cakes and wedding cakes.

Frosting ... is made from icing sugar and a fat such as milk or cream, often with added vanilla essence or cocoa powder for flavouring.

Rolled fondant icing ... is made from sugar and water to which lard which is whipped to introduce air bubbles can be added. The lard makes the icing lighter and more spreadable and so easier to lay or pipe.

It is used as a hard top covering for wedding cakes and similar cakes.

Marzipan ... is made from a mixture of sugar or honey and ground almonds (or plain almond paste).

It is used to provide a protective layer on top of fruit cakes before an external coat of white icing is applied.

All good stuff to be sampled at your peril. I have yet to find a cake that would not seriously interfere with my efforts to beat my diabetes.

22 - Legumes

Legumes are flowering plants. Many (but not all) legumes have edible seeds (called pulses). Pulses include beans, lentils, lupins (a type of bean), peas, peanuts, and soy beans.

Legumes have comparatively higher protein contents than other plants.

However, as I discovered when I started researching their nutritional values, they provide relatively low quantities of certain essential amino acids, such as acid methionine.

Balanced diet

There are many kinds of proteins but all of them consist of chains of amino acids. In fact, amino acids are the basic building blocks of proteins as they can be linked together in various sequences to form a vast range of proteins.

The human body is able to synthesize many amino acids from other compounds. However, there are nine amino acids ... the *essential amino acids* ... which you body must obtain as food because it cannot make them itself in sufficient quantities to maintain health.

According to the protein combining theory, in order to ensure you ingest adequate levels of the nine essential amino acids, you should combine legumes with other sources of protein in the same meal.

Vegetarian meals, for example, often combine a legume (such as beans) with grains to create a more complete protein than either legumes or grains on their own.

It seems to me that obtaining a balanced meal (one which delivers all nine essential amino acids) is a tricky business requiring an advanced understanding of nutrition, knowledge which I do not have. For this reason, I still eat some meat or fish in the hope that this will ensure that my diet is complete in respect of all essential amino acids.

Nevertheless, combining sources of protein is normal. Indians mix dal (lentils, peas or beans made into a stew) with rice. Mexicans stuff corn tortillas with beans. Foodies combine tofu with rice, while most Americans love smearing peanut butter on their wheat bread.

Protein combining seems to have lost favour among scientists in recent years, though I did not find any research that concluded that the theory is complete bunk. Nutritionists still believe that a variety of protein sources is healthy, but these do not have to be consumed at the same meal.

Health benefits of legumes

Pulses are good for you. They are high-protein foods with very low GIs, and are rich in calcium, iron and soluble fibre, and contain traces of good fats such as omega-3 fatty acids.

According to researchers at the University of Kentucky, people who eat legumes regularly are slimmer and have less LDL ('bad') cholesterol and more HDL cholesterol than people who don't eat legumes.

In my view, eating legumes in the form of pulses is essential for beating your diabetes, controlling your blood pressure and cholesterol, and maintaining a proper body weight. They can be the basis of many great dishes ... chickpea salad, black bean chilli ... and they make for hearty, healthy meals.

Here's what I discovered using internet research on some of the most popular and healthful pulses.

Beans

Beans are high in protein but very low in fat and have no cholesterol. They are full of complex carbohydrates, yet have a low GI, which means they are very helpful for controlling your glucose and cholesterol levels.

Beans also have high levels of folate, thiamine, vitamin B6, calcium, potassium, selenium, molybdenum and iron. They're pretty good all round.

Even better, this pulse also contains significant amounts of both insoluble and soluble fibre. One cup of cooked beans has between 9 and 13 grams of fibre, depending on the variety. This is one reason why people who eat beans often weight less than those who don't.

Indeed, a US government survey showed that those who eat beans regularly weigh 6.5lbs (3kg) less on average than non-bean-eaters, while bean-eating teenagers weight an average of 7lbs (3.2 kg) less and their waistlines are nearly an inch narrower than teens who don't eat beans. Regular bean-eaters also have lower levels of bad LDL cholesterol and higher levels of good HDL cholesterol.

When beans are growing they are encased in pods. Green beans are eaten whole. Others are shelled before they are eaten. The shelled beans can be eaten fresh or they can be dried for storage and then rehydrated for eating.

Green beans ... include string (runner) beans, stringless (French) beans, snap beans, wax beans, and some kidney beans. Compared to dry beans, green beans provide less starch and protein, and more vitamins A and C.

They can be steamed, boiled, stir-fried and added to casseroles.

Shelled beans ... include several types of kidney beans, pinto beans, and pea beans, among others. Fresh shell beans are nutritionally similar to dry beans, and are often steamed, fried, or made into soups.

Dried beans ... will keep indefinitely if stored in a cool, dry place but, as time passes, their nutritive value and flavour degrade and cooking times lengthen. They are almost always cooked by boiling, often after being soaked for several hours.

They can also be bought cooked and canned as whole beans with water, salt, and sometimes sugar or as refried beans (cooked and mashed beans). Tinned (canned) beans are just as good as dried beans as far as I know and save a lot of preparation time.

There are hundreds of varieties of beans ... black beans ... black turtle beans ... cranberry beans ... pinto beans ... flageolet beans ... pea beans ... navy bean ... cannellini ... fava (broad) beans... lima beans (aka butter or Madagascar beans) ... red kidney beans ... to name a few. If you like experimenting in the kitchen, there are enough beans out there to keep you busy for years.

While all beans are highly nutritious, some are better than others.

All beans are good for your heart. However, according to a study I found in the *Journal of Nutrition*, people who eat a 3-ounce serving of **black beans** a day decrease their risk of heart attack by 38 per cent. Black beans are also full of anthocyanins, antioxidant compounds that have been shown to improve brain function.

The **pinto bean** is the bean most commonly used for refried beans (fresh or canned). They can help reduce cholesterol levels. If you combine pinto beans with rice and serve the mixture with cornbread or corn tortillas, you'll have a balanced meal, as this combination contains all the essential amino acids.

You'll find pinto beans in chilli con carne, though other beans such as kidney beans or black beans may be used in this dish.

The small, white **navy bean** (aka pea bean or haricot) is for baked beans and bean pies. Scientists have shown that eating baked beans lowers both total and LDL ('bad') cholesterol levels.

This might be partly explained by the high levels of saponin (a chemical compound with anti-bacterial and anti-fungal properties) in navy beans. Saponins have been found to inhibit the growth of cancer cells.

Not all beans are safe to eat without some precautions being taken. For example, eating a few raw red kidney beans can cause vomiting and diarrhoea, due to a toxin called phytohaemagglutinin. This toxin must be deactivated by boiling for ten minutes at full blast (100 °C / 212 °F) before eating or cooking, even if the beans are going to be cooked for hours at a low heat, as in a slow cooker.

Flatulence from beans

Many beans contain oligosaccharides, a type of sugar molecule also found in cabbage. To digest these molecules properly, an anti-oligosaccharide enzyme is necessary but your digestive tract does not contain these, so oligosaccharides are digested in the large intestine by bacteria.

This results in gas as a by-product, hence the flatulence you get from eating beans.

In my experience, flatulence is especially troublesome when you first start eating beans regularly. However its severity diminishes gradually.

In the meantime, I discovered, there are plenty of things you can do to reduce the gas. You can, for example, cook beans with anise seeds, coriander seeds and cumin but, though this can be effective in reducing the output of gas, these spices do lend their own flavours to the food.

A good trick is to soak the beans overnight in alkaline water (which you can make by adding baking soda to ordinary water) and then rinsing thoroughly before cooking. If you soak with ordinary water, you should change it several times during soaking; and not use that water to cook the beans, as it will have absorbed some of the gas-producing sugars.

You can also add vinegar but only after the beans are cooked as vinegar interferes with the softening of the beans during cooking.

Tinned (canned) beans generate less gas than the beans you process yourself. This is because the canning process eliminates some of the gas-producing sugars. And, fermented beans will not usually produce a lot of gas either, as yeast can consume the offending sugars.

Cooking beans

Unless you stick to tinned (canned) beans, you will have to cook beans sometime. Beans take a long time to cook.

Dried legumes, with the exceptions of black-eyed peas and lentils, need to be rehydrated in water that's at room-temperature. Slow overnight soaking is best.

If you want to get rid of the indigestible sugars that cause flatulence, boil the beans for a few minutes and then set them aside overnight in the same water. When you through out the water in the morning it will contain most of the dissolved sugars.

After soaking, rinse the beans and put them in a pot with three times their volume of water. Add herbs or spices if you want. Bring to a boil. Then reduce the heat and simmer gently, uncovered, stirring occasionally, until tender. Add more water if the beans become uncovered.

The cooking time depends on the type of bean, but takes at least 45 minutes. Beans are done when they can be easily mashed between two fingers or with a fork.

I discovered that you can freeze cooked beans. Just immerse them in cold water to cool them and drain them well before freezing.

If you want to add salt or acidic ingredients, such as vinegar, tomatoes or juice, wait until the beans are just getting tender, near the end of the cooking time. If you add these too early, they can make the beans tough and slow the cooking down.

Peas

Peas are highly nutritious and very versatile. They are particularly high in fibre, protein, vitamins and minerals and thus will help you beat your diabetes. And they are not the boring old vegetable of our youth ... they can be used in an amazing range of cuisines and dishes.

Peas grow in pods. Each pod contains several peas. Most peas are immature when eaten, but a few varieties are grown to maturity and used to produce dry peas.

Peas do not keep well and need to be used quickly or preserved by drying, canning or freezing within a few hours of being picked.

Pod peas ... aka mange-tout or 'eat all', are eaten unshelled while still unripe. Compared to garden peas, the pod is less fibrous and therefore edible when the pea is young.

Pod peas do not open when they are ripe but mature peas may need stringing, ie have the string running along the top of the pod removed, before they are eaten. The pods will come apart if they are over-cooked.

Garden peas ... aka green peas, are peas that are harvested while they are still immature and are shelled and eaten immediately.

These are the peas most of us eat, whether fresh, frozen or tinned (canned). There are many different varieties. Most of the peas eaten in the West are garden peas.

Dried peas ... are usually field peas, ie peas that have been left to grow in the fields until they are mature instead of being harvested when they are young.

There are various kinds of dried peas and they can play a significant role in our diets.

Marrowfat peas ... are large, starchy, mature peas that have been allowed to dry out naturally in the field.

Mushy peas ... are marrowfat peas that have been steeped overnight in water before being simmered gently until they form a thick lumpy green soup, which is served with fish and chips.

Processed peas ... are mature peas that have been harvested, dried, soaked and then heat treated to prevent spoilage, similar to the pasteurisation of milk.

Split peas ... are peas that have been shelled, dried, peeled and split. Once the skin has been removed, the natural split in the seed can be used to separate the sections.

Because more surface area is exposed, split peas cook faster than other peas.

Peas are high in fibre (5g per 100g), protein (4 to 5g per 100g), vitamins, minerals and lutein. Pod peas in particular have plenty of vitamins A and C, iron and potassium, and they are low in sodium. They have virtually no fat, while total carbohydrates are between 12 and 14g per 100g.

Peas tend to spoil soon after they are harvested. However, they can be canned or frozen. Nutritionally, there seems to be little difference between raw fresh peas and frozen or canned peas.

Peas are usually boiled or steamed as this breaks down the cell walls, giving them a sweeter taste, and makes the nutrients more bio-available.

Most of the peas I have ever eaten have either been fresh peas from the garden, which we used to gather everyday in season when I was a child, or peas from a shop (fresh, frozen or canned). These have always been served as an accompaniment to a meal or as an ingredient in soup.`

It wasn't until I began researching peas to see if they could help me beat my diabetes that I realised how versatile peas are ... peas are eaten in hundreds of different ways around the world.

In Western cuisine, as well as accompanying a main course, peas are also used in casseroles, pies and salads. Pod peas are often stir-fried. In Indian cuisine, green peas are used in curries, while split peas are used to make dhal.

I've always been fond of pea soup which is made from dried peas. In the UK, dried yellow split peas are used to make pease pudding (pease porridge), which is similar to split pea soup in the USA. In the eastern Mediterranean, peas are made into a stew with meat and potatoes.

In China, the green shoots of snow peas (a pod pea) can be cut and served as a vegetable or stir-fried with garlic or shellfish. Snap peas (another type of pod pea) are eaten uncooked in salads, and can also be steamed or stir-fried.

Peas, I discovered, are even used in stand-alone snacks. Roasted and salted peas, for example, are sold as nibbles in Japan, China, Taiwan and Southeast Asian countries such as Thailand and Malaysia.

Chickpeas

Chickpeas are high in protein and fibre and are a great help in beating diabetes. They come disguised in a variety of names ... ceci bean ... garbanzo bean ... chana ... sanagalu Indian pea, and ... Bengal gram.

But there are only two main types: (a) the Desi and (b) the Kabuli.

The Desi chickpea has small, darkish seeds and a rough coat, while the Kabuli chickpea has lighter coloured, larger seeds and a smoother coat. Within each type there are several varieties.

The Desi has much more fibre and a lower glycemic index value than the Kabuli. Thus, to beat diabetes, you should choose Desi chickpeas.

Unfortunately, a distinction between Desi and Kabuli is not yet mandatory on the labels of tinned (canned) chickpeas, the most common source of this legume in the West.

Nevertheless, both types of chickpeas are very nutritious. A hundred grams of mature chickpeas, boiled without salt, contains about 164 calories, 2.6g of fat (of which only 0.27g is saturated), 7.6g of dietary fibre and 8.9g of protein.

Chickpeas also deliver plenty of vitamins A, B complex, C, E and K, as well calcium, iron, magnesium, phosphorus, potassium, and zinc. At the same time, they contain negligible amounts of sodium, about 7mg per 100g. Recent studies show that chickpeas can help lower blood cholesterol levels.

As you can see, getting chickpeas into your diet will be of enormous help in beating your diabetes. You can use them in all sorts of different dishes ... just add chickpeas to salads, soups, stews, pasta sauces and stir-fries. The tinned (canned) varieties are fine.

Up to recently I knew little about chickpeas, even though I had been eating them for years in Indian and Arabic food. Here's what I found out. The various uses of this legume are wondrous.

Chickpeas are a major source of protein in the (mainly) vegetarian culture of India, where they are used to make curries. Mature chickpeas are also ground into flour to make many popular dishes and snacks. Unripe chickpeas are also eaten raw as snacks, while the leaves are used in green salads.

In the Arab World, chickpea flour is shaped into balls and deep-fried as falafel. Chickpeas are also cooked, ground into a paste and mixed with sesame seed paste (tahina) to make hummus, as well as being roasted, spiced, and eaten as a snack.

In other parts of the world the flour is used as a batter to coat vegetables and meats before frying, to make fritters, patties and flatbreads. In the Philippines, garbanzo beans, a variety of chickpea, are preserved in syrup and eaten as sweets, and are used in desserts such as halo-halo. Some varieties of chickpeas can even be popped like popcorn and then eaten.

My favourite ways to eat chickpeas are in salads and hummus. For salads, I open a small tin (can) of pre-cooked chickpeas and mix them into a bowl of chopped lettuce, tomato, onion, peppers etc.

Hummus is great for beating your diabetes. The problem is that lots of commercial brands are too high in fat, though some low fat hummus is now available from major chains. However you can easily make your own with a food processor. You just cook the chickpeas and shove them into the blender, and add spices or flavourings as you like.

To make smooth hummus the cooked chickpeas must be processed while they are still quite hot, before the skins have had a chance to harden. Note also that dried chickpeas take one to two hours to cook properly but can easily fall apart if they are cooked for too long. If you soak them overnight (for 12–24 hours) first, the cooking time can be reduced to about half-an-hour.

Lentils

Lentils are high in nutritional value. A 100g of dry raw lentils contains 60g of carbohydrates (of which only 2g are sugars), just 1g of fat, and is rich in vitamins B1 and B9.

It also contains some calcium, more than half your daily requirement for iron, and about one-third of the magnesium, nearly two-thirds of the phosphorus, a fifth of the potassium and half the zinc that you need on a daily basis.

At the same time, lentils are a low calorie food ... only 230 calories in a whole cup of cooked lentils.

Dry raw lentils also contain about 26g of protein per 100g. This is extremely high, almost as good as soybeans. The proteins in lentils include the essential amino acids isoleucine and lysine.

But they lack two other essential amino acids, methionine and cysteine. You can overcome this shortfall by mixing lentils with grains (eg, rice) to create a complete protein dish, one with all the essential amino acids.

Sprouted lentils, however, contain all essential amino acids, including methionine and cysteine. You can sprout dried lentils by soaking them in water for a day and then keeping them moist for several days.

Lentils are a rich source of dietary fibre. But the amount available depends on the type of lentil. Red lentils, for example, only have 11% fibre, while green lentils contain about 31%. This fibre is both insoluble and soluble. Red lentils have a GI of 31, green lentils about 37, both extremely low.

Lentils are usually sold in pre-packed quantities. Before you buy you need to check for moisture or insect damage and make sure the lentils are whole and not cracked.

You should store lentils in an airtight container in a cool, dry and dark place. This way, they will keep for up to 12 months.

Lentils do not lose nutritional value when they are canned, but you need to read the label on the tin to ensure that the tin does not contain extra salt or other additives.

There are dozens of different types of lentils, which vary in size and colour. They are sold in many forms ... with or without the skins, whole or split.

They are relatively quick and easy to prepare and they absorb flavours easily from seasonings and other foods. Lentils are extremely popular. Cooked lentils can be used in stuffing because they are soft.

In the West they are most commonly consumed in lentil soup or in salads. In Egypt and Asia lentils are often combined with rice, which has a similar cooking time, to create a balanced meal.

Unlike other legumes, lentils do not need to be pre-soaked before cooking. But first you need to clean them thoroughly under cold running water.

To boil, use three cups of water to one of lentils.

To make them easier to digest, boil the water first, before putting in the lentils, rather than bringing the water to a boil with the lentils already inside.

When the water returns to the boil, turn down the heat, cover and allow them to simmer for anything from 10 to 40 minutes depending on the variety ... shorter for small varieties with the husk removed, such as the common red lentil.

The actual cooking time will also depend on what the lentils are for. If they are being cooked for a salad you'll need a firmer texture and should remove them from the heat 5 or 10 minutes early. You should also shorten the time if they are for a soup and will be cooked further with vegetables.

If you need a mushier consistency (eg, to make dhal), cook for an extra 10 to 15 minutes. Note that lentils with husks remain whole with moderate cooking, while de-husked lentils tend to disintegrate into a thick purée.

Caution ... lentils contain purines which can lead to excessive uric acid in the body, which can cause gout or kidney stones. If you are susceptible to these conditions, you should not eat too much lentil.

Peanuts

The peanut (aka groundnut, monkey nut, pigmy nut etc) is, despite its name and appearance, not a nut but a legume. Peanuts can be eaten raw, used in recipes, and made into peanut butter.

Because peanut butter is full of protein and resists spoiling for a long time, it is popular as a spread for bread. It is also used in the manufacture of sandwiches, sweets (candies) and bakery products.

Popular peanut snacks in the West, especially the Americas, include boiled peanuts, salted peanuts (which have usually been roasted in oil) and dry-roasted peanuts. Peanuts are cheaper than real nuts such as Brazil nuts, cashew nuts, etc, and so are used a lot in mixed nuts.

Peanut products include peanut butter sandwiches, peanut candy bars, peanut butter cookies, peanut brittle, etc, etc.

Peanuts are rich in nutrients, providing over 30 essential nutrients and non-essential phytonutrients. They contain about 25% protein, more than any real nut. They also have plenty of fibre (about 9%) and are a good source of niacin, folate, fibre, magnesium, vitamin E, manganese and phosphorus. They also are naturally free of trans-fats and sodium.

The problem for a diabetic is that a 100g of peanuts contains about 48g of fat, of which 7g is saturated, 24g monounsaturated, and 16g is polyunsaturated. For this reason I never eat peanuts, peanut butter or peanut snacks.

The only time I have peanuts is in a Thai or Chinese restaurant when, as an occasional indulgence, I will have a satay-type dish.

Soya beans and products

The Chinese have been eating soya beans (or soybeans to

Americans) for about 5,000 years. As a substitute for diary products, such as milk, soy can be a great help in helping you beat diabetes.

All raw soya beans are toxic and have to be cooked before they can be eaten. There are three kinds:

Green soya beans ... aka edamame beans, are young soya beans picked just before they ripen. You have to boil the pods lightly in salted water before you can eat the beans and throw away the empty pods.

You can buy both fresh and frozen edamame beans.

Mature soya-beans ... are harvested when they have reached maturity. These light brown soya-beans need to be kept in the refrigerator and used within a few days. To prepare them, you shell them and boil the beans until they are tender.

You can use mature soya-beans in salads, as a side dish for a main meal and as an ingredient in casseroles, stews and soups.

Dried soya-beans ... need to be soaked overnight before being boiled slowly. It takes three hours or so before they become tender. But you can buy pre-cooked soya beans in tins (cans).

However, eating soya beans will not help you beat your diabetes ... they contain about 20% fat! But many soya products can be a great help in beating diabetes as they are made from the 'de-fatted' remainder after the fat has been extracted for vegetable oil.

Protein accounts for about 40% of dry soya beans by weight. Most soy protein is relatively heat-stable and this stability allows soy food products requiring high temperature cooking, such as tofu, soy milk and textured vegetable protein, to be made.

Soya-beans are considered a source of complete protein, ie one that contains significant amounts of all the essential amino acids, and has been endorsed as a good source of protein by the US Food and Drug Administration.

Though it contains all the amino acids found in milk and meat, soya, not being an animal product, is low in saturated fats and is cholesterol free.

It is also rich in soluble fibre (9.3%) and high in the essential omega 3 fats. Raw mature soya-beans contain over 30% carbohydrates (including more than 7% sugars).

A 100g of these beans has 20g of fat (of which nearly 3g is saturated), which is why you have to check labels to make sure that soy products have been de-fatted.

Raw beans also contain vitamins A, B6, B12, C and K, and Choline (an essential nutrient required for the proper functioning of all cells).

Dietary minerals include calcium, iron, magnesium, phosphorus, potassium, sodium and zinc, while the beans also contain significant amounts of alpha-linolenic acid (omega-3) and isoflavones (which are antioxidants).

Most of us experience the soya bean as a food product, rather then by eating the beans as snacks, salads, or in soups or stews. These products include: soya-bean oil, soya meal, soya flour, textured vegetable protein (TVP), soy milk, tofu, tempeh, soy lecithin, and soy sauce.

Soya-bean oil ... is extracted from the soya-beans by first cracking the beans, adjusting for moisture content, and rolling into flakes, after which the oil is extracted using a solvent.

Soya-bean oil is often refined. Sometimes it is hydrogenated or partially hydrogenated. Soya-bean oils, including those that are partially hydrogenated, end up in a wide variety of processed foods.

Soya meal ... is what's left after the oil has been extracted from the soya-bean flakes, heat-treated and ground. Its protein content is 50%. It is processed into a range of food products.

Once the soy-bean meal has been ground finely, it is known as **soya flour** or **defatted soy flour** as it contains less than 1% fat. **Low-fat soy flour** is made by adding some oil back to the defatted flour.

Full-fat soy flour ... is made from de-hulled and ground beans that still have all their oil. It can also be made by adding soya-bean oil to defatted flour.

Textured vegetable protein

Soya flour is used to make textured vegetable protein (TVP), aka textured soy protein (TSP) or soya meat, which can be used as a replacement for meat in many recipes.

Because the soya bean oil has been taken out, TVP is very low in fat and is a good source of fibre and protein. It has no flavour of its own but because of its sponge like texture, it soaks up flavours well. TVP can soak up to three times its weight in liquids and is quick cooking.

It comes in dried chunks, nuggets, flakes, grains and mince, to which you have to add water to use it in a recipe.

TVP can contain as much as 50% protein when dry. It is usually rehydrated using two units of water to one of TVP, which reduces protein to 16% or so, about the same as mince (ground) meat. And, of course, it does not have the fat and cholesterol associated with meat.

Textured vegetable protein is a versatile substance. It is used to make vegetarian versions of meat dishes such as chilli, spaghetti Bolognese, burgers, tacos and burritos.

But you should check the labels of burgers and sausages made from TVP for fat content, as fat is added during manufacturing.

Personally I am not at all fond of TVP chunks. I don't like their texture and feel that they don't absorb flavours as much as everyone says.

But I am rather fond of the mince type of TVP and rather enjoy using it to thicken up a meat sauce such as Bolognese ... when cooked with meat it absorbs the juices (and therefore flavours) that would usually be lost.

Soy milk
Soy milk is a traditional staple of Chinese and Japanese cuisines. It is opaque, white or off-white in colour, and has the same consistency as cow's milk. I am very fond of soy milk and use it daily.

Soy milk is made from dry whole soya beans or full-fat soya flour. The beans are soaked in water for at least three hours, usually overnight. Once rehydrated, they are 'wet ground', ie ground finely in about ten times their own weight of water, and the resulting mush is boiled for about 20 minutes. After this the 'milk' is filtered to remove the insoluble residue (soya pulp fibre).

Plain soy milk has about 3.5% proteins (the same as cow's milk, though the actual amino acids are different). It only contains about 2% fat (less than full-fat cow's milk) and no cholesterol. Soy milk also has just over 6% carbohydrates of which 4% are sugars, and perhaps 0.5% dietary fibre. It gives you plenty of B vitamins, some vitamin E, and copious amounts of dietary minerals.

However much of the mineral content in soy milk is unassimilable because it is high in phytic acid, which makes some minor minerals (such as zinc and iron) unabsorbable, as well as to a lesser extent macro-minerals such as calcium and magnesium. For this reason, soy milk may be fortified with calcium and other minerals, as well as with vitamins D2, B12 and B2.

Soy milk is found in many vegan and vegetarian food products and can be used as a replacement for cow's milk in many recipes. I use it in my coffee and in my breakfast porridge. Provided it still has some fat in it, its taste is very palatable.

Soy milk is processed to create further soy products. Its coagulated protein can be made into tofu by curdling and draining, just as dairy milk is made into cheese. Soy milk is used to make soy yogurt, soy cream, soy kefir (fermented milk) and soy-based cheese analogues.

Soy milk skin ... is used in Japanese and Chinese cooking. It is made by boiling soy milk in a shallow open pan, which results in a film or skin made up mainly of protein and fat appearing on the surface. The film is dried into yellowish sheets containing about 52% protein, 25% fat, and 12% carbohydrate.

Okara ... aka soy pulp or tofu lees, is the fibre, protein, and starch left over when the milk has been extracted from the soybeans. In the West it is often put into vegetarian burgers.

Soy cheese ... is made from soya beans and vegetable oils. There are many different varieties, from cheddar style to mozzarella to soft spreadable cheeses. They are usually full of fat so the advice is, if you are serious about beating your diabetes, to ignore them. I certainly do.

Soy yoghurt ... is made using soy milk and yoghurt bacteria. Some soy yoghurts are deliciously tart but I would advise caution ... sometimes sweeteners, such as fructose, glucose, or raw sugar, are added. Again, as always, check the labels.

Tofu

Tofu (aka bean curd) is the most commonly used soya product. It is made by clotting soy milk using a coagulant and then pressing the curds into soft white blocks.

There are two main types: fresh tofu, which is produced from soy milk, and processed tofu, which is made by processing fresh tofu further.

Fresh tofu ... comes in three main types. They differ in the amount of water taken from the curds.
Silken tofu contains the highest moisture content. It's like very fine custard and you eat it with a spoon.
Firm tofu contains less water. It's like firm custard and can be picked up with chopsticks.
Chinese dry tofu contains the least moisture though it has not actually been dried. It feels rubbery.

Flavours such as fruit acids can be mixed directly into soy milk prior to curdling. **Sweet dessert tofus**, such as almond mango, coconut or longan tofus, have the texture of silken tofu and are served cold.

Processed tofu ... comes in many guises.
Pickled or preserved tofu consists of cubes of dried tofu that have been allowed to dry and ferment slowly in the open air.
Stinky tofu is an aptly named soft tofu that has been fermented in a salt-water mix of vegetable and fish brine ... the least said the better.

Tofu has a low calorie count, relatively large amounts of protein (by weight, about 10.7% for firm tofu and 5.3% for silken tofu), and little fat (5% for firm tofu and 2% for silken tofu).

It is high in iron and may be high in calcium and/or magnesium depending on the coagulant used to make it.

But it is fairly flavourless and can be used in both savoury and sweet dishes as a bland background for presenting the flavours of other ingredients.

Tofu is often marinated in soy sauce, or with chillies and sesame oil. Silken tofu is used in sweet dishes, sauces, dips and spreads. Firm tofu can be fried, deep fried, sautéed, roasted and stir-fried.

Tofu can also be preserved by freezing.

In the West, tofu is often used as a substitute for meat, while many tofu dishes in Asia include meat. Indeed tofu is eaten ... raw, stewed or stir-fried, in soup, cooked in sauce, or stuffed with fillings.

I must admit that I am somewhat partial to sweet or dessert tofus. The problem is, they often have lots of added sugar so you need to be careful and read the labelling closely.

I'm not so fond of tofu in savoury dishes. It's ok in a dip or as a substitute for egg in a quiche ... but only ok. Where it shines for me is as bean curd (another name for tofu) in Chinese or Thai cuisine in, for example, dishes containing black beans or sweet and sour sauces.

Tempeh (soy cake)

Tempeh is a traditional Indonesian food made by fermenting cooked soya beans using a Rhizopus mould as a starter. Fermentation binds the soya beans into a patty, similar to a firm vegetarian burger. Other grains, such as barley, may be added, as well as spices and various flavourings.

You can make tempeh at home using whole soya beans. If the beans are still in their hulls, you need to soften them by soaking before you can de-hull them. Then soak the de-hulled beans overnight before cooking them for about 30 minutes.

After that, you mix in a tempeh starter and spread the beans out in a thin layer in a warm room (at about 30 degrees C). Fermentation will bind the softened beans together and within 48 hours you'll have a fresh cake of tempeh.

Tempeh has a different texture and better nutritional characteristics than tofu. It has more protein and vitamins. As it contains eight out of nine of the essential amino acids, tempeh is almost a complete protein food. It also gains additional digestive benefits from the enzymes formed during fermentation.

Fermentation makes the soy carbohydrates in tempeh more digestible. In Asia, the starter-culture used often contains bacteria that produce vitamins such as B12. In western countries, however, a pure culture that makes very little B12 is more common.

Fermentation also reduces the phytic acid in soy, which in turn allows the body to absorb the minerals that soy provides.

Depending on the brand, 100g of tempeh provides around 200 calories, 18.2 grams of protein (more than tofu), no cholesterol, and plenty of calcium and iron. However if also contains 11g of fat of which 2g is saturated. Indeed over 45% of its calories come from fat.

Tempeh has a firm texture and a nutty mushroom-like flavour which becomes more pronounced as it ages. This contrasts very favourably with tofu's bland texture and lack of flavour. And it is very versatile and can be used in many different ways.

Normally tempeh is sliced or cut in cubes and fried (often after being marinated) until the surface is crisp and golden brown, while the inside stays soft.

Cooked tempeh can be eaten on its own, or used in chilli, stir-fries, soups, stews, salads, and sandwiches. It freezes well. You can also grate it like cheese and used grated tempeh instead of minced (ground) beef in tacos or Bolognese sauce.

Tempeh is, admittedly, a bit of an acquired taste but I like it. It wasn't fond of it at first but then it grew on me. Maybe I'm a persistent fellow. However, I am also a pretty cautious dude and, because of the fat it contains, eat only a little tempeh.

Miso
Miso is a traditional Japanese seasoning produced by fermenting soya beans (sometimes with barley or rice) with salt and a special fungus. The result is a thick paste used for sauces and spreads, pickling vegetables or meats, and for flavouring soup.

The flavour and aroma depends on the ingredients and the length of fermentation. High in protein, vitamins and minerals, miso is very nutritious as it also contains soy protein and isoflavones. The problem for those with metabolic syndrome is that it is high in salt, which is evident from the taste.

Miso is sold as a paste in a sealed container and must be refrigerated after opening. It contains many beneficial micro-organisms which can be killed by over-cooking. Thus it is best to add miso to soups or other foods just before they are removed from the heat, or to use it without any cooking at all.

The only time I eat is miso is when I have miso soup, a traditional Japanese soup made by mixing softened miso paste into a stock. I buy instant miso soup in single-serving packs which have a shelf-life of up to a year. These usually contain dried wakame (a type of seaweed) and tofu with soy beans that reconstitute rapidly when hot water is added. It's got a tart taste that I have grown to like a lot.

Soy sauce
Soy sauce is a salty brownish liquid that has been used in cooking

and as a condiment in East and Southeast Asian cuisines for thousands of years.

It is made by fermenting soya beans (with a grain, such as wheat) using moulds, salt and water. The resulting paste is pressed to extract the sauce and the cake that's left is used as animal feed. Soy sauces made in various regions differ in smell, taste and saltiness.

Soy sauce is now quite common in Western cuisine, even though it does not contain the level of isoflavones associated with other soy products such as tofu or edamame.

The main problem for those of us who have metabolic syndrome is that soy sauce contains up to 18% salt ... a total no-no if you are trying to control your blood pressure and beat your diabetes.

Even low-sodium soy sauces contain too much sodium because it is virtually impossible to produce soy sauce without using some salt.

In addition, the UK Food Standards Agency has found carcinogens in some brands of soy sauce made in mainland China, Taiwan, Hong Kong, Thailand and Vietnam in recent years. This is another reason why I avoid soy sauce almost entirely, except as an occasional flavour-enhancer in cooking.

23 - Vegetables and fruit

We all know that eating vegetables and fruit is good for you ... whether you are a diabetic or not.

For healthy people, a diet in which vegetables and fruit predominate may (provided the rest of their diet is good) reduce their risk of heart disease and stroke, protect against some cancers and, due to a low calorie count and the presence of dietary fibre, reduce the risk they will become obese or develop type 2 diabetes.

The potassium in vegetables and fruit can also help lower blood pressure, reduce bone loss due to aging, and reduce the risk of developing kidney stones.

For you and me, making vegetables and fruit a core part of our diet is vital to beating our diabetes, something I realised early on when I was told that they are nearly all very low in fat. Indeed I was an enthusiastic eater of vegetables and fruit and had my diabetes pretty much under control before I began to do detailed research on this core part of my diet.

What's the difference?

Most of us know the difference between a vegetable and a fruit ... or rather we think we do ... so imagine my surprise when I found out that the botanical definitions don't always agree with the everyday use of these two words.

To a botanist, a vegetable is an edible plant or edible part of a plant, such as a leaf, stem or root, while a fruit is an edible part that has developed from the ovary of a flowering plant ... it includes many poisonous fruits no chef would dream of using.

Many plants we usually view as vegetables (such as eggplants, bell peppers, and tomatoes) are fruits in botany. And a mushroom, which most of us consider a vegetable, is not even a plant ... it's a fungus!

For me, I'm gonna stick to the usual use of the terms in Western kitchens ... a fruit is any edible part of a plant that has a sweet flavour and a vegetable is any edible part with a savoury flavour.

Hygiene

As with all foods, vegetables and fruit can become contaminated and spread diseases. Thus, for safe eating, they require proper preparation and handling. You probably know most of what I'm about to discuss here but to me, a renowned domestic incompetent, much of it was a (surprising) revelation.

Safety begins at the selection stage. When choosing fresh vegetables and fruit, check them carefully to make sure they are not damaged or bruised.

You should also rinse all vegetable and fruit before preparing them or eating them raw. This even applies to fruit that will be peeled. To avoid spoilage, the cleaning should be done immediately before the produce is prepared or eaten.

Vegetables and fruit should be stored separately from raw animal foods such as meat, poultry, and seafood. They should also be kept clear of any surfaces (eg, cutting boards) and utensils that have been used to prepare animal foods. In fact, if vegetables and fruit have touched raw meat, poultry, eggs, or seafood, they should be thrown away unless they are going to be cooked soon.

Because it does not take long for harmful bacteria to grow on vegetables and fruit that have been peeled, cut or cooked, they should be put in a refrigerator as soon as possible.

Most vegetables should be stored in the vegetable drawer of the refrigerator. The exceptions are vegetables such as potatoes, onions, and garlic which should be placed in ventilated containers and stored separately in a cool dark place.

Greens should be thoroughly dry before storage, lest they turn slimy. Unused bits of cut onions can be stored in the refrigerator.

All vegetables should be stored away from fruits ... fruits give off ethylene gas as they ripen, which causes any vegetables near them to decay rapidly.

Dried herbs and spices should be stored in glass jars or bottles in a dark cupboard. The labels on the containers should be dated and dried herbs should not be kept for more than three or four months.

Preserving vitamins during cooking

When you are boiling food, water-soluble vitamins, such as vitamins C and B, can be washed out into the water. To prevent this you should use as little water as possible and cook the food (usually vegetables) for as short a time as possible. You can then save and reuse the cooking water in other foods (eg, soups) so as not to lose those vitamins.

Even better ... eat your vegetables and fruit raw and you won't risk losing any vitamins. I do this and have found immense enjoyment in preparing and eating a wide variety of fresh mixed salads.

Eat locally grown produce

Advances in agricultural and food-handling technology, as well as transportation, means that most fruits and vegetables are mass produced and harvested in a steady year-round stream of produce which can be distributed to consumers half a world away.

This makes for greater availability of fresh, uniformly-sized vegetables and fruit, and it seems nowadays that certain produce is never out of season.

While mass-produced vegetables and fruit may be perfectly healthy to eat, there are several good reasons why I opt for locally grown produce from small farmers, gardeners and orchard keepers.

Mechanical growing and handling methods, and the rigours of long distance transport, mean that large-scale commercial growers are more concerned with the hardiness of their produce and care less about its flavour and texture. As a result, the vegetables and fruit in your local supermarket do not usually have the same taste as produce that's grown locally.

In addition, produce that's grown on small-scale farms, gardens and orchards is usually organically grown, ie without the use of artificial fertiliser, which means it contains less toxins and is probably more nutritious.

24 - Vegetables

There are literally hundreds of vegetables you can eat. Most are nutritious and a great help in beating diabetes.

Nearly all vegetables are low in fat and none have any cholesterol. They usually have fewer calories per serving than other foods, which is helpful if you need to lose weight.

Vegetables also have low GIs, with the exception of potatoes. All vegetables contain dietary fibre, some more than others.

There are plenty of vitamins in vegetables but the actual vitamins and quantities vary from vegetable to vegetable. Vegetables also contain *provitamins* (substances that are converted to vitamins within the body) and dietary minerals, all of which again vary widely depending on the particular vegetable.

Vegetables also contain a great variety of other *phytochemicals* (chemicals found in plants that are useful but are not essential nutrients). Some of these are said to have antioxidant, antiviral, antibacterial, antifungal and anti-carcinogenic properties.

We usually eat vegetables as part of our main meals. You can also eat them as snacks, either cooked or raw. However, some vegetables must be cooked to make them edible, and there are usually eaten as part of savoury dishes. A few vegetables are used in sweet foods or desserts, such as carrot cake and rhubarb pie.

Ketchup, tomato sauce and vegetable oils are some of the processed foods derived from vegetables. These may not contain all the nutrition of the vegetables used to make them. They may also contain additives such as sugar that diabetics must avoid. Read the labels.

Fresh, frozen or canned

Personally I enjoy vegetables immensely and find eating them very satisfying.

But my big question has always been: what is the difference in nutrition (if any) between fresh, frozen and canned vegetables?

Here's what I found out courtesy of Mr Google.

Vegetables are at their nutritious best just after they have been picked. In addition, tests show that frozen vegetables are just as nutritious as fresh ones. However, if they are frozen immediately after being picked, they may be more nutritious than 'fresh' vegetables that are eaten several days after being harvested (ie, that are shop-bought rather being from your own garden).

Frozen vegetables are also more convenient ... all you need to do is to steam them a bit and they are ready.

Canned or tinned vegetables, however, have lower nutritional values than fresh or frozen. This is because the best way to preserve the nutritional content of vegetables is to cook them lightly for a short period of time (ie, eat them al-dente rather than as a soggy mush), and canning requires a long cooking time at higher temperatures.

How much to eat

Most dietary guidelines recommend at least five servings of vegetables or fruit a day, one serving being half a cup of either raw or cooked vegetables, though for leafy greens, such as lettuce and spinach, a single serving is one cup.

I don't find this recommendation convincing at all. The concept of 'servings' bears no relationship to nutritional content (which is what matters) and the nutrients they contain vary widely between different vegetables.

It's also fairly irrelevant.

If you follow the sort of diet I am using to beat my diabetes ... a plant-focused diet in which vegetables are the main dish and meat is the side-dish ... you will be eating more than enough vegetables to maintain your health and enjoy your food.

Classifying vegetables by parts eaten

When we eat vegetables, we seldom eat the whole of the plant, just one part, eg, the roots, leaves, stems or seeds ... and vegetables can be classified by the part of the plant we usually eat. The remarkable thing is that many of the vegetables grouped this way have similar nutrients.

Here's what I found out:

Leafy vegetables ... include salad greens (such as lettuce), spinach, collard greens, kale, bak choy, leeks and watercress. Some leafy greens (eg, turnip greens and beet greens) are the tops of root vegetables which are also edible.

Leafy vegetables, such as salad greens, are eaten raw. Others, such as kale and collard greens, are usually cooked, but can also be consumed raw.

Most leafy vegetables are rich in carotenoids (such as beta carotene), vitamin C and folate. They also provide chlorophyll, iron, and calcium in varying amounts, and are good sources of fibre.

Flowers, buds, and stalks ... range from celery, through broccoli, cauliflower, asparagus, Brussels sprouts, artichokes, rhubarb, Chinese celery, to bamboo shoots and capers.

As most of these have their own flavours they are usually eaten plain. However they are sometimes served in sauces or other flavoursome liquids which can, unfortunately, contain plenty of fat or sugar.

Most of these vegetables are great sources of vitamin C, calcium, and potassium. They also provide a plenty of dietary fibre. Broccoli and cauliflower are said to contain cancer-fighting compounds.

Roots, bulbs, and tubers ... are vegetables that grow underground. They include onions, shallots, garlic, turnips, potatoes, Jerusalem artichokes, sweet potatoes, taro, yams, beets, carrots, radishes, and parsnips.

These vegetables are dense and satisfying to eat. However their nutritional content can vary. For example, potatoes are good sources of vitamin C and potassium, while radishes and turnips also deliver fibre, and sweet potatoes and carrots deliver lots of beta carotene. In some cases, the tops of these vegetables (such as beet greens and scallions) contain more nutrients than the roots or bulbs.

Some studies suggest that onions and garlic may lower blood pressure and cholesterol levels.

Due to their high starch content many of these vegetables contain more calories than most above-ground vegetables and can trigger rapid rises in blood glucose. However, as they are packed full of nutrients, they should be eaten but only in moderation.

Fruit vegetables ... include peppers, tomatoes, cucumbers, squash, zucchinis, pumpkins, peppers, eggplants, okra (lady fingers), breadfruit and avocado. Botanically speaking, these are all fruits because they are the fleshy parts of plants and contain seeds.

However, they are used as vegetables.

Most fruit vegetables are higher in calories than leafy vegetables, stalks, or flowers. They are also good sources of vitamin C. As they offer a variety of flavours and textures that blend well with many dishes, so you can use them as extra ingredients in stews and soups.

Colour and nutrients

Another useful way to classify vegetables is by their colour, which is usually a good indicator of nutritional content.

For example, green vegetables (spinach, cabbage, asparagus, broccoli, kale, Swiss chard, etc) have plenty of iron and, except for spinach, calcium. Orange vegetables (carrots, yams, butternut squash, etc) are full of beta-carotene, which fights cancer.

So colour can be a handy way for deciding which vegetables to put on your plate.

Or you can list vegetables according to their nutrients. You get potassium (which helps control blood pressure) from sweet potatoes, white potatoes, spinach, legumes, and tomato products (paste, sauce, and juice).

But creating such a list would require an in-depth knowledge of all vegetables. Just going by colour would likely be nearly as good.

Vegetables for beating diabetes

Most vegetables contain the complex carbohydrates that provide energy. They also supply dietary fibre and the vitamins and minerals needed for good health. In fact, vegetables are nutrient dense, ie compared to the small amount of calories they contain their level of nutrients is high.

This makes them the cornerstone of a diet for beating diabetes.

Consuming a variety of raw vegetables is a great way to get an adequate supply of plant food nutrition. This is because, although all vegetables will have several nutrients in common, if you compare two vegetables, you are likely to find that each of them has nutrients that the other does not have. It seems that different vegetables have been designed to complement each other.

To combine vegetables on a plate so the nutrients in each individual vegetable complement the nutrients in the other vegetables would require the sort of list mentioned above. As this is likely to be very lengthy, it would be difficult to manage.

However, during my research on the internet, I discovered an easier way which can be fairly useful in matching complementary vegetables ... combining different colours.

As already mentioned, colour is a good clue to the nutrient content of vegetables. For example, most yellow and orange vegetables (eg, carrots and sweet potatoes) get their colour from their high content of beta carotene and other carotenoids, ie substances the body turns into vitamin A.

Dark-green leafy vegetables contain high levels of chlorophyll, the green pigment that enables plants to absorb energy from light. Chlorophyll is a natural blood purifier and is nutrient dense. It helps stabilise the body's acid-alkaline balance, remove unwanted residues and activate enzymes. It may have a role in preventing liver, skin and colon cancers.

Chlorophyll is most abundant in green leafy vegetables, such as spinach, lettuce and members of the cabbage family.

Thus, so long as your plate contains some yellow or orange vegetables plus some green leafy ones you are probably getting all the nutrients you need for health. But there is another little-known substance you need to check for: choline.

Choline is a water-soluble essential nutrient, a newly discovered B vitamin. It is used to synthesise certain components in cell membranes and must be consumed through food if your body is to remain healthy.

So you need to make sure you consume vegetables that contain choline on a regular basis. These include iceberg lettuce, spinach, cauliflower and other members of the cabbage family.

Raw vegetables are a better source of vegetable nutrients than cooked vegetables. Most of us eat raw vegetables in salads. However, modern kitchen appliances have made turning raw vegetables into juices and smoothies very easy. Their high levels of nutrients and low levels of natural sugars mean that vegetables can be the main ingredients in liquid foods.

Drinking raw freshly-pressed vegetable juice is a great source of nutrition. The best raw juices consist mainly of vegetables to which a compatible fruit (such as apples) has been added.

Colours can be very useful when inventing juices ... add a non-green vegetable (such as carrots) and/or a fruit (such as apples) to a green juice to create a drink with a balance of nutrients.

Raw vegetables can be consumed as green smoothies, made up of a mix of green leafy vegetables and sweet fruits. For me, the best taste is got by mixing a mildly-flavoured leafy vegetable (such as spinach or lettuce) with a tropical fruit that contains little water (such as a banana or mango).

Of course, you should try other vegetable-fruit combinations ... experimentation is the game here.

Choosing vegetables

All vegetables, with very few exceptions, are full of vitamins and other nutrients. So how do you decide what to buy from the vast range on offer in your local supermarket?

It's a tough choice. But here's what I pick and why ... based on how useful these vegetables are in beating diabetes.

Tomatoes

Tomatoes are low in calories and are packed with nutrition, especially when they are fully ripe. I eat at least one tomato a day ... every day ... no exceptions.

How ripe a tomato is makes a difference in terms of nutrition. Red tomatoes, for example, contain up to four times the amount of beta-carotene as green tomatoes.

One of these beta-carotenes is lycopene. Studies have shown that lycopene neutralises harmful oxygen-free radicals before they can damage the structures of your cells, protecting you against various cancers.

Tomatoes are even more beneficial for those of us who have both diabetes and metabolic syndrome ... they reduce our cholesterol levels, thus lowering our risks of heart disease, cataracts, and macular degeneration.

If you can't get fresh tomatoes, don't worry. Cooked tomatoes and processed tomatoes (such as tomato paste) are just as good. Indeed cooking makes it easier for the body to absorb the lycopene, so cooked tomatoes may be better. But there's always a risk that nutrients will be compromised by cooking, which is why I always eat a fresh tomato as well as tomatoes included in cooked dishes.

Cabbage family

In my daily meal, I also include a vegetable from the cabbage family (aka the crucifers or cruciferous vegetables) ... cabbage ... Brussels sprouts ... broccoli ... cauliflower ... turnips ... kale ... bok choy ... rapeseed, and ... radishes.

Some of these vegetables are eaten as leaves or greens (eg, cabbages), others as roots (eg, turnips). Either way, they deliver all the nutrients you need to beat your diabetes.

They are excellent sources of vitamins B6 and C, and also have plenty of vitamins B1, B2, and E, as well as manganese and carotenes. Greens in the cabbage family also deliver plenty of fibre, iron, copper, and calcium.

In fact cruciferous vegetables have much higher levels of calcium than they do of phosphorus. This is important because phosphorus reduces the utilization of calcium. So that calcium can do its job of keeping your bones healthy, you need to ingest more calcium than phosphorus. As the greens in the cabbage family contain almost three times more calcium than phosphorus, anyone with a family history of osteoporosis should eat them (especially bok choy) regularly.

These vegetables are also good for you in other ways. Turnips, for example, have only about one-third of the calories of ordinary potatoes, while broccoli is one of the most nutrient-dense foods you can find.

Crucifers also seem to have anti-cancer properties. Statistics show that the higher the intake of these vegetables, the lower the rates of breast, lung, colon, and prostate cancers and for these reasons the American Cancer Society recommends eating crucifers on a regular basis.

Carrots

Among all the vegetables we normally eat, carrots have the highest quantities of carotenes which the body turns into vitamin A ... which I why I include them in my food as often as possible.

Carrots are good for your vision. Their beta-carotene helps protect against macular degeneration (a major worry for diabetics) and the development of cataracts.

Carrots also enhance your looks. Their copious amounts of vitamin A prevent the production of too many cells in the outer layer of your skin which means, with fewer dead cells, you get a clearer skin.

Carrots are also full of carotenoids, fat-soluble compounds associated with a reduced risk of a wide range of cancers, cardiovascular disease, asthma and rheumatoid arthritis.

A high intake of carotene has been linked with a 20% decrease in postmenopausal breast cancer and up to a 50% decrease in cancers of the cervix, bladder, colon, prostate, larynx, and oesophagus. Extensive studies have shown that a diet that includes at least one carrot per day could cut the rate of lung cancer in half.

Artichokes

Artichokes are not easy to come by where I live, but I get them whenever I can. Why? Because this vegetable helps improve my blood glucose and cholesterol levels, among other good things.

Fresh artichokes contain carbohydrate in the form of inulin, a starch the body handles differently than other sugars and which has been shown to improve blood glucose control in diabetes.

This vegetable also protects the liver from damage by promoting the flow of bile and fat to and from that organ. And they lower cholesterol levels by increasing the excretion of cholesterol and decreasing its manufacture in the liver.

Artichokes also contain antioxidants that cut the risk of stroke.

Celery

For those of us with metabolic syndrome (ie, 85% of all type 2 diabetics), celery should be a vegetable of choice. It can help lower blood pressure and cholesterol levels.

The ability of celery to help lower blood pressure is due to the coumarins and potassium it contains. *Coumarins* are phytochemicals that tone the vascular system, lowering blood pressure. They also enhance the activity of certain white blood cells and are said to be effective in preventing cancer.

Most plant foods provide some potassium, but only two (celery and bananas) contain very high levels of it. The potassium in celery is well-balanced with the other minerals and nutrients that the vegetable provides.

Studies have also shown that celery may help lower cholesterol.

The problem with celery is that it is really not very tasty. However, as an ingredient in juice it works well because of its high water content ... try a refreshing celery and apple combo. In fact, because potassium is an electrolyte, drinking celery-based juices after a workout is great for replacing electrolytes lost through sweating.

Spinach

I've always liked spinach. It is one of the most nutrient-dense vegetables, supplying copious amounts of vitamins and minerals. It is also one of the most alkaline of foods and helps regulate the body's pH balance.

Spinach is also one of the richest dietary sources of lutein, an antioxidant that may help to hinder arteries from getting clogged. Thus, it is effective in promoting healthy eye sight and preventing macular degeneration and cataracts, always a worry for diabetics.

The chlorophyll and carotene in spinach have anticancer properties. Spinach contains at least 13 different flavonoids that function as antioxidants and anticancer agents.

In addition, its vitamins and nutrients can bolster bone-mineral density, attack prostate cancer cells, reduce the risk of skin tumours, fight colon cancer, and, last but not least if you are a man, increase blood flow to the penis.

Boiled gently with shredded onion, spinach makes a great tasting, ultra-healthy side-dish.

Lettuce

All lettuce is a good source of vitamin K and chlorophyll, though this is not the main reason I eat these leaves several times a week. For me it is the basis of a great salad. And any time I make up a sandwich, I always include a layer of lettuce.

As lettuce is very low in calories and high in water, it's very useful when trying to lose weight. But different varieties of lettuce differ in the nutrients they contain. The Romaine variety is the most nutrient-dense, while iceberg lettuce is a good source of choline.

Potatoes, sweet potatoes and yams

There's nothing wrong with ordinary (white) potatoes ... their skins are full of vitamins, minerals and fibre, and they deliver a fairly decent amount of protein.

The drawback with potatoes is that they have a relatively high GI value compared to other vegetables. For this reasons, I tend to use sweet potatoes or yams instead of potatoes.

Sweet potatoes are one of the healthiest foods on Earth. They are excellent sources of carotenes; the darker they are the more they contain. They also contain plenty of vitamins and dietary minerals.

Their proteins contain glutathione, an antioxidant that can enhance the metabolism of nutrients and the health of the immune-system, and also protect against a wide range of diseases. Sweet potatoes are also said to counter the effects of second-hand smoke.

Unlike many other starchy vegetables, their low GI value ensures that sweet potatoes are a great diabetes beater and a wondrous substitute for ordinary potatoes.

Yams too have very low GI values and, with similar properties to sweet potatoes, also make a great substitute for ordinary potatoes.

Peppers

Bell peppers are low in calories and very nutrient-dense. As a diabetic, you'll be pleased to know that, due to beta-carotene, they are effective in protecting against cataracts.

Bell peppers also contain some powerful phytochemicals which deliver exceptional antioxidant activity. They also contain substances that prevent the formation of blood clots and reduce the risk of heart attacks and strokes.

Not all peppers are the same. Red bell peppers have much more nutrients than green peppers. Red bells also contain lycopene, a carotene that offers protection against cancer and heart disease. Both sorts, however, are great in salads, stews, casseroles and stir-fries.

Onions and garlic

I try to eat onions and garlic as much as possible. These two pungent roots can be of immense help in controlling diabetes and tackling metabolic syndrome.

Studies have shown that onions help lower blood glucose levels significantly, while onions, onion extracts and garlic lower blood pressure and prevent the formation of blood clots.

Garlic decreases total cholesterol levels while increasing levels of HDL ('good') cholesterol. Studies also show that garlic protects against atherosclerosis and heart disease.

Pretty good survival stuff!

Mushrooms

I always try to eat mushrooms at least twice a week for several good reasons:

Though raw edible mushrooms don't contain any vitamin C or sodium, they are a good source of B vitamins and essential minerals. As they are low in fat, carbohydrate and calories, and fibre makes up 8 to 10 percent of their dry weight, they are ideal for losing weight.

All the many varieties of mushrooms are excellent sources of potassium, which helps lower blood pressure and reduces the risk of stroke. One serving of mushrooms also provides 20 to 40 percent of you daily need for copper, which has cardio-protective properties.

Mushrooms are a rich source of selenium, an antioxidant that cuts the risk of prostrate cancer significantly. White button mushrooms can reduce the risk of breast cancer and prostate cancer.

Reiki, shiitake, and maitake mushrooms are rich in an antioxidant that protects cells from abnormal growth and replication, ie, reduces the risk of cancer ... cooking them in red wine which contains resveratrol is said to magnify their immunity-boosting power.

In addition, shiitake mushrooms seem to stimulate the immune system and fight infections, and have been used for centuries in China and Japan to treat colds and flu.

Other vegetables

There are many other vegetables which I enjoy on a regular basis.

I also like eating asparagus (protein rich and great in salads), leeks (which can improve the immune system, lower bad cholesterol levels and support sexual functioning), eggplants (also cholesterol lowering), and squashes.

There are so many different vegetables out there that we are spoiled for choice. Try a different vegetable every week. You'll be surprised at what you may discover.

Vegetables I avoid

There are two vegetables I avoid completely ... avocados and olives. The reason? They are both full of fat, the killer for persons with type 2 diabetes.

Avocados ... are highly nutritious. Unfortunately about 20% of an avocado is fat, and even though it is mainly unsaturated, it is still fat. In fact, the oils contained in avocados include oleic and linoleic acids which are reputed to help to lower cholesterol levels.

No matter, these fats will still block the receptors in your muscle cells which, as you have type 2 diabetes, you are trying to unplug with your diet. Avocados, therefore, are strictly off my menu. I can get all the omega-3 and-6 I want from supplements.

Olives ... also have a very high fat content, between 15 to 35 percent depending on the variety. The fat in olive oil is 'good' fat, and indeed people in the Mediterranean area who consume large amounts of olive oil are less likely to develop diabetes than Americans or Northern Europeans.

The problem is ... you have already developed diabetes, and to beat your diabetes you need to focus on unblocking those muscle receptors. For this simple reason olives too are off the table.

Choosing vegetables

Except for roots, bulbs and tubers, vegetables can start to go rotten fairly quickly so, when buying, you need to select only the freshest. Check for mould and only select vegetables that feel crisp and have vivid colours.

Leafy vegetables should be crisp and moist, with strong colours. If they look yellowish, they are probably wilting, ie beginning to rot. If the leafs have tiny holes, insects have been at work.

Check flower, bud, and stalk vegetables carefully. The leaves on flower vegetables should be bright green and fresh-looking. The florets on cauliflower and broccoli should be tightly closed and evenly coloured and they should not have a strong smell. Stems should be firm and crisp without any slime. Ripe artichokes feel heavy for their size and squeak when squeezed.

Roots (such as beets, carrots, and turnips) should be smooth, hard, and free of bruises and cuts, with bright colours. The leaves of root vegetables should be crisp and vivid green with no yellow spots.

Carrots should be reddish-orange, not pale or yellow ... the darker the orange, the more the beta carotene. The top may be tinged with green, but dark green or black on the top indicates decay. In fact the green part on the top is bitter and should be cut off before eating.

Potatoes should feel firm, have a uniform colour and be free of sprouts. Sprouting means the potato has started to age and contains increased amounts of solanine (a naturally-occurring toxin). Any eyes (the buds from which sprouts grow) should be few and shallow. The skins should be smooth and dry and should not be green-looking, which would mean that solanine if building up. To stop them turning green, store potatoes away from light.

Fruit vegetables should be plump and smooth, with no bruises. Any leaves should be fresh and green-looking.

25 - Fruit

There are hundreds of fruits you can eat and most of them are delicious, whether they are eaten whole, cut-up into pieces or pureed. You can buy them fresh, canned, frozen or dried.

Fruits lend themselves to various forms of processing. They are pressed to make fruit juices, are preserved as jams and marmalades, or used to make alcoholic beverages and vinegars. Fruits are also found in products such as biscuits (cookies), muffins, yogurts, ice creams, cakes and desserts.

Nutritional values

Fruits are good for you ... very, very good for you. You couldn't eat better. They are full of vitamins, especially vitamin C, and dietary minerals and contain no animal fat or cholesterol.

Most fruits are high in fibre and nearly all (except for watermelons and pineapples) have low GIs.

Fruits also contain sugars. The amount varies widely between different fruits. Lime, for example, only has traces of sugar while sugar makes up over 60% of the weight of fresh dates.

Fruits also contain various *phytochemicals*. These are chemicals that are beneficial but not essential nutrients which you get from eating plants. However, research indicates that phytochemicals are required for the long-term health of cells and the prevention of disease.

In sum, fruits provide excellent nutrition. And here are a few more facts I discovered when trawling the internet:

(1) Frozen fruits are, nutritionally-speaking, the equivalent of fresh but they are more convenient.

(2) Dried fruits also have low GIs, just like fresh fruits, but as the water has been removed, you tend to eat more of them than fresh fruits.

(3) Regular consumption of fruit is associated with reduced risks of cancer, cardiovascular disease (especially coronary heart disease), stroke, Alzheimer disease, cataracts, and some of the functional declines associated with aging.

(4) Diets that include a sufficient amount of potassium from fruits and vegetables also help reduce the chance of developing kidney stones and may help reduce the effects of bone-loss.

(5) Fruits are low in calories so they can be useful for losing weight.

How much to eat

I was always told in the diabetes clinics I attended to limit my consumption of fruit to a maximum of three pieces a day ... eg, one banana, one apple and half a glass of pure fruit juice ... because of the natural sugars contained in all fruits.

However, most fruit (with a few exceptions) have low GIs and so their sugars are released slowly into the bloodstream and do not cause a spike in blood glucose levels. When I discovered this fact, I began to ignore the conventional advice about limiting my intake of fruit with no adverse effects.

My personal view is that there are too many good things in fruit to risk missing out, so I don't limit the amount of fruit I eat. In fact, I feel that the three pieces of fruit a day should be a minimum rather than a maximum.

All fruits are good for you. However there are some fruits that, despite their low GIs, contain too much sugar for a type 2 diabetic. In addition, some fruit may interfere with the actions of some of the medicines you are taking. Here's what I came up with on the internet for some popular fruits.

Apple

Apples contain very little fat or protein, and a reasonable amount of dietary fibre (2.4%), though less than other fruits. However their total carbohydrate content is about 14% of which more than 10% is sugars.

But, as they have a GI of 38, which means that glucose will be released fairly slowly into your blood-stream, you can eat them, even though like me you are a diabetic, provided you don't over-indulge.

Compared to many other fruits and vegetables, apples contain relatively low amounts of vitamin C. But they are a rich source of other antioxidants that prevent damage to cells. Research suggests (but does not prove) that apples may reduce the risk of colon cancer, prostate cancer and lung cancer.

An apple a day is said to reduce swellings of all kinds, due to quercetin, a flavonoid which reduces the risk of allergies, heart attack, Alzheimer's, Parkinson's, and prostate and lung cancers.

In addition, apple juice and apple juice concentrate have been found to increase the production of the neurotransmitter acetylcholine in mice and thereby reduce cognitive decline due to aging.

You can eat the whole of a fresh apple, including the skin. Indeed it is best to eat the skin as it contains many of the micro-nutrients.

However the core should not be eaten as the seeds in the centre are mildly poisonous. They contain a small amount of amygdalin, a cyanogenic glycoside, though usually not enough to be dangerous to humans.

Some brands of apple juice have added sugar, so check the ingredients. Personally I prefer to stick to fresh apples ... I eat one a day in the afternoon as a snack.

Pear

Pears have no fat and very little protein. However they contain over 15% carbohydrates of which sugars make up nearly 10%. Pears, though, have a similar GI to apples (35 to 40 depending on the variety) so they can be eaten with care by diabetics.

Pears have plenty of vitamin C and fibre (3.1% by weight), both of which are found mainly within the skin. Most of the fibre is insoluble, making pears a good laxative. But you have to eat the skins.

Pears ripen at room temperature. They ripen faster if you place them next to bananas in a fruit bowl. Refrigeration slows ripening and adds two or three days to their shelf life. Pears ripen from the inside out and are ripe when the flesh around the stem-end or neck gives to gentle pressure.

A ripe pear is sweet and juicy, and a joy to eat. I use them as a substitute for my daily apple now and then.

Apricots

Apricots contain no cholesterol, virtually no fat and very little sodium. A 100g delivers about 1.4g of protein. They are a good source of dietary fibre and potassium, and a very good source of vitamin A and vitamin C ... 100g provides 2g of fibre, 1.9g of potassium, 96µg of vitamin A, 1094µg of beta-carotene and 10mg of vitamin C.

But, with total carbohydrates of 11g per 100g, a large portion of the calories in this food come from sugars (9g per 100g). At 57, the GI of fresh apricots is not as low as other fruits so diabetics need to exercise caution. However dried apricots have a GI of 32 or so and thus would be a preferred choice.

Indeed, dried apricots have greater nutritional value overall than fresh ones because all the nutrients are concentrated. As all the water has been removed, the ratio of fibre to the volume of fruit is high for dried apricots. This means that you can use dried apricots to relieve constipation ... you'll probably feel the effect after eating just three or so.

If you are taking a diuretic, which is likely if you are controlling your blood pressure using medications, you will need to continuously replace the potassium you lose in your urine. Apricots can be a handy and effective potassium-replacer.

However, I noticed that there is some dissention among nutritionists as to whether the form of potassium found in apricots (potassium gluconate) is absorbed by the body as easily as other forms such as potassium citrate or potassium chloride.

Peach and nectarine

Peaches and nectarines belong to the same species. The difference is that peaches have a fuzzy skin while the skin of nectarines is smooth. Nectarines are also a bit smaller and sweeter than peaches.

Peaches and nectarines have no cholesterol and virtually no fat or sodium. A 100g contains less than 1g of protein. However they are a reasonable source of dietary fibre (about 1.5g per 100g), vitamin A, niacin and potassium, and a very good source of vitamin C (6.6mg per 100g).

But a large portion of the calories come from sugars. Indeed 100g contains nearly 8.5g of sugars. Considering that the GI of peaches can be as high as 56 and nectarines usually have a GI of 43, diabetics (that's you and me) need to exercise restraint when eating peaches or nectarines.

Peaches and nectarines are climacteric, ie they continue to ripen after being picked. Store them at room temperature, however, as putting them in the refrigerator gives them a more bland taste.

Cherry

This fleshy stone fruit is sugar heavy. Total carbohydrates are 16g per 100g, of which 13g consists of sugars. However, as they have a

GI of 22, cherries can probably be eaten in moderation by diabetics.

Cherries are very low in fat and sodium, and contain about 1.1g of protein per 100g. They are also a good source of dietary fibre (2g per 100g) and vitamin C (7mg).

Cherries are also said to confer benefits beyond the merely nutritional. They contain anthocyanins, potent antioxidants that are currently being researched. Cherry anthocyanins have been shown to reduce pain and inflammation in rats.

In addition, studies sponsored by the Cherry Marketing Institute suggest that cherries may reduce the risks of getting heart disease or diabetes but I could not find any independent confirmation of these claims on the internet.

Plums and prunes

Fresh plums have a waxy coating on their skin which reduces the loss of moisture but which can be rubbed off easily. Dried plums are called prunes.

There are hundreds of varieties of plums ... damson, greengage, yellowgage or golden plum, Satsuma and Victoria being the best known ... each with its own distinct taste and colour. All can be dried.

A raw fresh plum (without its stone) has very little fat, protein or sodium. It is a good source of fibre (1.4g per 100g of fruit), vitamins A and K, phosphorus and potassium, and a very good source of vitamin C (9.5mg per 100g).

Unfortunately, 100g of plum has just 10g of sugars and, as its GI can be as high as 53 (and as low as 24) depending on the variety, diabetics should only eat it in strict moderation.

Drying a plum removes nearly all the water, so the nutritional value of a prune is dramatically different. The amount of vitamin C per 100g drops to 0.6mg (from 9.5mg), while the amounts of phosphorus and potassium more than quadruple. Prunes are also rich in copper and boron, both of which can help prevent osteoporosis.

Drying increases dietary fibre five fold to 7.1g per 100g. This fibre includes inulin which, when broken down by intestinal bacteria, makes a more acid environment in the digestive tract which, in turn, makes it easier for calcium to be absorbed.

Prunes contain total carbohydrates of 63.88g per 100g, of which 38.13g is sugars, ie the sugars in a prune are nearly four times the amounts in a fresh raw plum. Even though prunes have a GI value of only 29, they need to be treated with caution by diabetics. In fact, my advice would be to ignore them unless you need them for their laxative effects.

Indeed, both fresh plums and prunes have a well-know laxative effect, and prunes and prune juice are often used to help regulate the functioning of the digestive system.

Berries
GI values can only be calculated for foods containing sugar or starch. Certain foods, such as many berries, are high in fibre and very low in starch, so a GI value cannot be calculated.

Blackberry
Blackberries are notable for their high nutritional content, and I drop a few defrosted blackberries, along with other berries, into my porridge every the morning.

You'll get 5g of dietary fibre from 100g of raw blackberries, much more than from many other fruits. With 21mg of vitamin C and 20µg of vitamin K, 100g of blackberries will give you at least a fifth of you daily requirements of these two vitamins.

The same amount of the berries also contains 0.6mg of manganese, nearly 30% of your daily need for this essential mineral.

Blackberries also rank highly for the strength of their antioxidants, which include polyphenol antioxidants, naturally occurring chemicals that can have a beneficial effect on metabolic processes.

They are very low in fat and sodium. They have lots of large seeds that contain oil which is rich in omega-3 and -6 fats. Blackberries are also a good source of vitamin E (1.17mg per 100g), magnesium, potassium and copper.

Total carbohydrates are nearly 10g per 100g, of which sugar is only 5g, much less than other fruit, which makes blackberries a fairly good bet for diabetics even though GI figures are not available.

Raspberry
There are many types of raspberries, including red, black and purple raspberries. Red raspberries have been crossed with other species to produce hybrids. The loganberry, for example, is a cross between a raspberry and a blackberry.

As well as having a great taste raspberries are nutritionally excellent and are always part of the mixed berries I put into my porridge in the morning.

Raspberries are a rich source of vitamin C ... 100g contains about 26mg, about a third of your daily needs. These berries also contain considerable quantities of vitamins B1, B2 and B3, folic acid, magnesium, copper, iron and manganese.

They also deliver significant amounts of polyphenol antioxidants and, like blackberries, rank very highly for antioxidant strength.

The GI of raspberries is not measurable. However the dietary fibre in raspberries can run from 8 to 20 percent per total weight. This means that even though they contain over 5g of sugars per 100g of fruit, they will probably release glucose into your blood-stream slowly.

Blueberry

I like the taste of blueberries and was adding two tablespoons to my porridge each morning before I found out how good they are for me.

Blueberries are very low in fat and sodium. But total carbohydrates are 14.5g out of 100g, of which a bit over 10g consists of sugars. Blueberries, however, also contain 2.4% dietary fibre which suggests that the rate at which glucose is released is fairly moderate and that small amounts can be eaten by diabetics.

Blueberries deliver a diverse range of micronutrients. Eating 100g will give you about 8% (0.1mg) of your daily requirement for B6, 12% (10mg) of the vitamin C you require and 18% (19µg) of vitamin K, as well as 14% (0.3mg) of the manganese you need daily.

Blueberries have a reputation for preventing certain medical conditions. They have been linked to a reduced risk of prostate cancer. Studies have also suggested that blueberries may be effective in reducing the risk of heart disease, type 2 diabetes and age-related memory loss in men.

The effects of consuming blueberries have been tested on animals. Feeding blueberries to rats was found to alter some vascular cell components that affect control of blood pressure. In other studies of animals the consumption of blueberries lowered cholesterol and total blood lipid levels.

It has been suggested that supplementing diets with wild blueberry juice may affect memory and learning in older adults, while reducing blood sugar and symptoms of depression.

Cranberry

Cranberries are related to blueberries. They have a sour, bitter taste ... I'm probably one of the few people who like eating them raw ... and are nearly always processed into products such as fruit juices, cranberry sauce, jams and dried cranberries.

The fresh fruit, however, can be used to add tartness to savoury dishes.

To reduce its tartness, cranberry juice is usually sweetened heavily or blended with other fruit juices, and you need to read the labels carefully before deciding to buy. Dried cranberries are invariably sweetened and should be avoided by diabetics.

Raw cranberries have moderate levels of vitamin C, dietary fibre and the essential dietary mineral manganese, as well as a balanced profile of other essential micronutrients. However, a 100g contains 12.2g of carbohydrates of which sugars are only 4g or so.

So, although the GI of cranberry is not available, the fruit should be OK for diabetics to eat in moderation, provided you don't add sugar. Hope you like the tart bitter taste.

Strawberry

Strawberries are an excellent source of vitamin C (57mg per 100g, ie, nearly the whole of your daily requirement) and manganese (29mg per 100g, ie, much more than your daily requirement).

They are also a very good source of folate (25μg per 100g), dietary fibre (2.3g per 100g) and iodine. Iodine is vital for keeping your thyroid healthy. Strawberries are also a good source of potassium, omega-3 fatty acids, magnesium, and vitamin K. They also contain a variety of phytonutrients, flavonols, hydroxycinnamic acids, and stilbenes.

However, 100g of strawberries contains just over 7g of carbohydrate, of which near 5g is sugar. But, as the GL of strawberries is 40, I feel that as a diabetic I can eat them in moderation.

Blackcurrant

Blackcurrants contain extraordinarily high levels of vitamin C ... 181–250mg in 100g, ie two to three times your daily requirement in a cup. They also contain good levels of potassium (322mg or 7% of your daily requirement in 100g), phosphorus (59mg or 8%), iron (1.5mg or 12%) and vitamin B5 (0.398mg or 8%), as well as a broad range of other essential nutrients.

Raw blackcurrants have the sort of strong, tart flavour I love and I enjoy eating them raw or dropping them into my porridge in the morning. But it seems that my tastes are not enjoyed by the population at large and the manufacturers of blackcurrant products ... juices, cordials, jams, jellies, sorbets, ice creams, yogurts, cheesecakes etc ... load them up with sugar.

I have yet to find a suitable blackcurrant product for diabetics. My advice is to forgo the juices and other products, and develop a liking for the raw blackcurrant. It really is delicious.

Try dropping a large spoonful into sauces, meat dishes and desserts ... you'll be surprised at the kick they give the flavours. And, if you hanker after a really refreshing tasty juice, blend some apples and blackcurrants together in a juicer but don't add any sugar. Savour it slowly to let the flavours dance across your taste buds.

Redcurrant

The redcurrant is nutritionally less well endowed than the blackcurrant, with only 41mg of vitamin C (about 50% of your daily requirements) per 100g. Levels of other micronutrients are also less than in blackcurrants, potassium (275mg or 6% of your daily requirement in 100g), phosphorus (44mg or 6%), iron (1mg or 8%) and vitamin B5 (0.064mg or 1%).

Nevertheless, redcurrants are a highly nutritious fruit and I always drop a few into my porridge in the morning.

The problem is the same as with blackcurrants ... sugar in redcurrant products, such as redcurrant sauce and redcurrant jelly, all of which are made by boiling redcurrants with sugar. All to be avoided by diabetics, that's you and me.

Gooseberry

Gooseberries are rich in vitamin C, 100g delivering around 40mg (45% of your daily requirements) and dietary fibre (about 4g per 100g). They are also good sources of vitamin A, potassium and manganese.

Whether eaten raw or cooked (without sugar), gooseberries have a brilliantly sharp taste. Another great thing about them is that their vitamin C is locked in, ie the quantity of vitamin C is not reduced by cooking.

Like blackcurrant and redcurrant products, gooseberry products ...

desserts, pies, jams, pickles etc ... contain oodles of sugar, so the advice is to shun them and concentrate on the plain goose-gob, raw or cooked. But the fruit is seasonal, so you can only get it at certain times of the year.

This is a pity because there is some evidence that eating gooseberries can help you control your diabetes by stimulating your body to produce insulin, which may help if your diabetes is advanced and your pancreas is not longer making enough of it.

You can, of course, freeze raw gooseberries. But the berries tend to collapse when they are thawed and the fruit goes all mushy ... however they are still all right for cooking.

Dates

Dates provide a wide range of essential nutrients. A 100g contains 2.45g of protein and 8g of dietary fibre ... regular eaters of dates seldom suffer from constipation.

Dates are also particularly rich in the B vitamins. A 100g contains 0.165mg of B6 (about 13% of your daily requirements), 0.589mg of B5 (12%), 1.274mg of B3 (8%), 0.066mg of B2 (6%), 0.052mg of B1 (5%), and 19μg of B9 (5%).

Dates contain plenty of trace elements. A 100g delivers, among other dietary minerals, 656mg of potassium (14% of your daily requirements), 43mg of magnesium (12%), 0.262mg of manganese (12%), 62mg of phosphorus (9%), and 1.02mg of iron (8%).

Unlike most fruits, dates contain little water (only about 20%) and so they do not become much more concentrated when they are dried. However, the small amount of vitamin C in dates is lost during drying.

Obviously, eating dates will supply you with plenty of nutrition. The problem is the sugar content ... 63% of ripe dates consists of sugars. The glycemic indices for the three different varieties of soft, semi-dry, and dry dates are 35.5, 49.7 and 30.5, which suggests that diabetics can eat a few dates but with caution.

However beware of stuffed dates and glazed dates.

Figs

Figs are highly nutritious. In fact, dried common figs are the richest plant sources of dietary fibre, copper, manganese, magnesium, potassium, and calcium relative to human needs.

About 10% of a fig, fresh or dried, consists of fibre and figs have a well-founded reputation as a laxative. The fibre in figs is also said to lower insulin and blood glucose levels.

Figs contain almost as much B vitamins as dates ... 100g delivers 0.434mg of B5 (about 9% of your daily requirements), 0.106mg of B6 (8%), 0.085mg of B1 (7%), and 0.082mg of B2 (7%). Like dates, they contain little vitamin C. But figs have plenty of antioxidants.

Figs are also packed with dietary minerals. Indeed, 100g contains 68mg of magnesium (19%), 162mg of calcium (16%), 2.03mg of iron (16%), 680mg of potassium (14%), 67mg of phosphorus (10%), and 0.55mg of zinc (6%).

Again as with dates, the problem is sugar. A 100g of figs contains nearly 64g of carbohydrates, of which sugars make up 48g. This is somewhat less than dates but nevertheless it means that figs have to be treated with caution by diabetics. I eat very few. If you take a risk and do eat figs, go the ones with dark skins, as they are the most nutritious.

Once they have been picked, figs do not keep well. Neither do they travel well. So obtaining fresh figs can be difficult and most figs are eaten dried or as a jam. There seems to be few nutritional differences between fresh and dried figs.

Grapes

Grapes, whether purple or green, contain no fat, very little protein and less than 1% dietary fibre. However they are very good sources of vitamins C and K, 100g of grapes providing about 13% of your daily requirements for vitamin C (10.8mg) and 21% of your daily requirements of vitamin K (22µg).

Grapes are also quite good sources of vitamins B1, B2 and B6, a 100g delivering 0.069mg (6%), 0.07mg (6%), and 0.086 mg (7%) respectively.

The problem, again, is sugar. Total carbohydrates are about 18g, of which sugars are 15.5g in a 100g of table grapes, ie raw grapes for eating. The GI of raw grapes is less than 50 so grapes should be OK in moderation for a diabetic provided you don't eat too many of them in one session.

Eating grapes and drinking a glass of red wine a day is said to be very good for you because all grapes contain large amounts of resveratrol, a polyphenol antioxidant which has been positively linked to inhibiting cancers, heart disease, degenerative nerve disease, viral infections and the mechanisms that lead to Alzheimer's disease, primarily in their skins and seeds.

The quantity varies between varieties. Fresh grape skin contains from 50 to 100mg of resveratrol per gram. White wine contains little resveratrol as (unlike red wine) it is not fermented with the skins. In fact, many nutritionists recommend a daily glass of red wine as, besides the resveratrol, the alcohol will dilate or widen your blood vessels, increasing the flow of blood and reducing blood pressure.

Pomegranate
The pomegranate is a delicious fruit to eat. It is very popular in the Middle East and other Eastern countries but in the West pomegranates are usually ingested in the form of juice.

Pomegranates are packed with vitamins and minerals. Indeed, a 100g of pomegranate will supply 12% of your daily need for vitamin C (10mg), 10% of the B3 (38µg) you need, 8% of the B5 (0.38mg), and about 6% each of the B1 (0.07mg) and B6 (0.08mg) you need.

The same amount of the fruit will also deliver 36mg of phosphorus (5% of your daily needs) and 236mg of potassium (5%) and 0.35mg of zinc (4% of your daily needs).

The problem, as always, is sugar. Total carbohydrates in 100g are 18.7g, of which 13.7g are sugars and 4g is dietary fibre. The GI for pomegranates is not available, ie we don't know how quickly the sugars are released into the blood-stream, so the fruit needs to be eaten with caution by diabetics.

A 100ml serving of pomegranate juice provides about 16% of an adult's daily vitamin C requirement, and is a good source of vitamin B5, potassium and natural phenols.

But the juice contains no fibre, which in the fruit is wholly contained in the edible seeds which are discarded to make the juice.

Commercially produced pomegranate juice has a GI of about 53. But as pomegranate juice is usually mixed with other fruit juices such as blueberries, the GI of will vary from brand to brand.

Pomegranates are considered a 'super-food' because of the polyphenols and antioxidants they contain. Indeed preliminary studies indicate that pomegranate juice may play a role in reducing the risk of cancer, reducing cholesterol levels and protecting arteries from getting clogged.

The juice has also been found to reduce systolic blood pressure and inhibit viral infections.

While the positive effects on cholesterol levels and blood

pressure can only be welcomed by those of us who have metabolic syndrome, some of these studies have been rather small and large independent clinical trials are needed to validate these findings.

Whatever the believable benefits are, they need to be balanced against the high sugar content of the juice.

Personally I like the taste of pomegranates (an intriguing mix of sweet and sour) and drink half a small glass in the morning when taking my supplements before breakfast.

Citrus fruits

Oranges, lemons, grapefruits and limes are the best known of the citrus fruits. Citrus fruits also include citrons, clementines, kumquats, mandarins, pomelos and tangerine among many others.

All citrus fruits have similar properties, and are a rich source of vitamins, minerals and dietary fibre. They also contain phytochemicals (biologically active, non-nutrient compounds) that can help to reduce the risk of many chronic diseases.

Citrus fruits contain no fat, no sodium and no cholesterol. The number of calories is low so they can be useful for reducing weight. These fruits also contain simple carbohydrates (fructose, glucose and sucrose) and citric acid.

All citrus fruit and unsweetened citrus peel have a low GI (less than 55) … the sharper the taste, the lower the GI … and so diabetics can eat them in moderation.

By eating citrus fruits you also get plenty of fibre (of which 65 to 70% is pectin). One medium-sized orange, for example, delivers 3g of fibre or 10% of the recommended daily intake of 25 to 30g.

Citrus fruits are great sources of vitamin C. A medium-sized lemon, for example, contains about 30mg of vitamin C, and a slightly larger one about 44mg. Indeed you can get up to 4mg of vitamin C from a slice of lemon. A lime gives you about 19mg of vitamin C. One medium-sized orange provides about 70mg of vitamin C, a naval orange about 82mg, and a large orange about 98mg, while a 225ml glass of orange juice contains approximately 125mg of vitamin C. And you'll get about 32mg of vitamin C from a large tangerine or mandarin orange.

Besides vitamin C, citrus fruits contain plenty of other vitamins such as thiamine (B1), Riboflavin (B2), niacin (B3), pantothenic acid (B5), vitamin B6 and folate (B9). A 225ml glass of orange juice, for example, delivers 75mcg of folic acid, more than a third of the recommended daily intake.

Citrus fruits are also rich in dietary minerals such as potassium, calcium, phosphorus, magnesium and copper. One medium orange provides about 235mg of potassium, while one 225ml glass of orange juice delivers 500mg of potassium, about a quarter of your daily requirement of 2,000mg.

There is considerable evidence that the phytochemicals in citrus fruits help reduce the risk or retard the progression of several serious disorders, several of which are of crucial importance to diabetics with metabolic syndrome … cardiovascular disease, heart disease, hypertension, stroke, cancer, and anaemia.

However not all citrus fruits are wholly beneficial, especially if you are taking certain medications. Grapefruit, for example, inhibits the enzymes that metabolize several medications in your intestines. This increases the concentration of these medications in your blood to levels that could be toxic.

These medicines include drugs for lowering cholesterol (such as atorvastatin (Lipitor), simvastatin (Zocor) and lovastatin (Mevacor)) and for controlling blood pressure (such as amlodipine (Norvasc), nifedipine (Adalat, Procardia) and verapamil (Isoptin, Calan)). Grapefruit also blocks the action of antihistamines and some psychiatric medications such as diazepam (Valium).

The effect lasts for 24 hours or more.

As I am taking statins to control my cholesterol levels, I never touch grapefruit. I understand that medical scientists are currently trying to find out whether other citrus fruits, such as oranges, have this effect but have yet to come up with conclusive answers. Thus I seldom eat oranges or other citrus fruits despite the tonnes of micro-nutrients they contain.

Guava
Guavas are rich in dietary fibre, vitamins C, B9 and A, as well as potassium, copper and manganese, though the actual amounts of micro-nutrients varies depending on the particular variety.

The fruit is especially rich in vitamin C. One guava fruit contains about four times the amount of vitamin C found in an orange. One serving of guava delivers 100% of your total vitamin C daily requirement.

The phytochemicals in guavas include both carotenoids and polyphenols, and the fruit's potential antioxidant value is relatively high compared to most plant foods. As these pigments are responsible for the colour of the fruit, red-orange guavas are better sources of polyphenols, carotenoids and pro-vitamin A than the yellow-green fruits.

Açaí

The skin and pulp of the açaí fruit contains lots of phenomenal properties. The carbohydrates in a 100g come to 52.2g but this includes 44.2g of dietary fibre and little sugar (as the pulp is not sweet).

However that 100g includes 32.5g of total fat. Açaí also contains many polyphenols.

Açaí is sold as frozen pulp or juice. It is also an ingredient in drinks, smoothies and foods. Over the last ten years spurious marketing hype has made it very popular as a supplement.

Did you know that açaí and its antioxidant qualities provide a variety of health benefits ... it can reverse diabetes (despite being 32% fat) and other chronic illnesses, as well as expanding the size of your penis and increasing your sexual virility if you are a male. It also promotes weight loss (without gender bias) and can help you control your weight.

Miracle stuff ... except that, unfortunately, there are no scientifically controlled independent studies that prove the fabulous health benefits you'll get from consuming açaí.

As far as I can tell, no açaí products have been officially evaluated by any reputable laboratory or research institution any where in the world.

And if the obviously false hype is not enough to put you off, just think of the fat content seemingly custom-designed to re-clog the receptors in your muscle cells!

Bananas

Bananas are climactic fruit, ie they mature on the tree but ripen off the tree. Green not-so-ripe bananas taste less sweet than yellow riper bananas because the latter contain more sugar and less starch than the former.

Bananas are picked when they are green and transported in low-temperature containers. Once they reach their markets they are ripened in air-tight rooms filled with ethylene gas. The vivid yellow you see on supermarket bananas is due to this artificial ripening process.

If your bananas are too green, putting them in a brown paper bag with an apple or a tomato will speed up the ripening process.

About one-eight of a ripe banana consists of sugars so, as you are a diabetic, you need to eat them with care. Bananas have a reasonable amount of soluble fibre (2.5g per 100g). A 100g of banana contains 8.7mg of vitamin C, about 10% of your daily requirement. The same weight of banana also delivers 0.3mg of manganese (14% of your daily requirement) and 358mg of potassium (8%).

The amount of potassium is less than I expected as I had been told by my medical advisor that I should eat one banana a day as I was low in potassium. I have since discovered that other fruits are more copious sources of potassium and that banana has relatively a lot of sugar. Nevertheless I still put one chopped banana into my porridge every morning.

Coconut

Coconut meat, the white stuff from inside the coconut, contains less sugar and more protein than bananas, apples and oranges. It is an excellent source of fibre and is relatively high in minerals such as iron, phosphorus and zinc.

A 100g of coconut meat contains 15.23g of carbohydrates of which only 6.23g is sugar and 9g is dietary fibre (one-third of your daily requirement). It also contains 3g of protein. It is a relative poor source of vitamins but a 100g does deliver 2.43mg of iron (19% of your daily requirements), 113mg of phosphorus (16%) and 1.1mg of zinc (12%).

The problem with eating coconut is fat ... a whopping 33.5g per 100g ... of which 30g or about 90% is saturated. As a diabetic aiming to beat your diabetes, you just need to forget about coconut. But it's OK to use it in shampoo.

Melon (White Antibes or Honeydew)

This kind of melon is a good source of vitamins B6 and B9 and potassium. It is an excellent source of vitamin C ... 100g contains 18mg of vitamin C, about a fifth of your daily requirements.

The only problem is that a 100g contains 9g of carbohydrate of which 8g is sugar. Therefore in your efforts to beat your diabetes you need to treat melon with caution.

Watermelon

A watermelon is about 92% water and 6% sugars by weight. It contains very little dietary fibre. However it is a good source of vitamin C ... 100g contains 8.1mg of vitamin C, about 10% of your daily requirements.

Watermelon has been shown to be mildly diuretic, ie it increases the flow of your urine. Some research suggests that watermelon may be useful in helping you reduce your blood pressure but, as far as I am aware, this still has to be proved under rigorous scientific conditions.

Kiwifruit

Though 100g of kiwifruit contains about 9g of sugar, it also has 3g of dietary fibre giving it a mildly laxative effect.

The same quantity of the fruit also delivers 0.63mg of B6 (about 48% of your dietary requirements), 40.3µg of vitamin K (38%) and 1.5mg of vitamin E. This quantity also gives you 92.7mg of vitamin C, more than a 100% of your daily requirement for vitamin C. Kiwifruit contains a fair bit of potassium, just slightly less than a banana.

All good stuff ... however a raw kiwifruit contains actinidin, an enzyme that dissolves protein, which is used to tenderise meat. Some people however are allergic to actinidin. In addition, raw kiwifruit should not be used in desserts containing milk or other dairy products as the actinidin will digest the milk proteins.

However it's OK to use cooked kiwifruit in these kinds of desserts.

Kiwifruit is considered by some scientists to be a natural blood thinner and can have effects that are similar to slow-release aspirin therapy.

Papaya

The ripe fruit of the papaya is usually eaten raw, with or without the skin or seeds. The unripe fruit can be cooked by being added to curries and stews, or can be added to salads after cooking.

A 100g of raw papaya contains nearly 10g of carbohydrates of which nearly 6g is sugar and less than 2g is dietary fibre. However, the same quantity also contains 328µg of vitamin A (about 41% of your daily requirements), 38µg of vitamin B9 (10%), 0.1mg of vitamin B6 (8%), and a massive 61.8mg of vitamin C (74%).

The skin, seeds and pulp also contain many phytochemicals including natural phenols.

Dried fruit

Dried fruit is fresh fruit from which most of the water has been removed.

Most of the nutritive value of the fresh is preserved, yet the dried fruit has a sweeter taste and a much longer shelf-life.

Fruit can be dried in two ways. The traditional method is either in the sun or in special heated wind tunnels.

The second way is to infuse the fruit with a sweetener (such as sucrose syrup) before drying, a method used to dry fruits such as cranberries, blueberries, cherries, strawberries and mangoes. Note that some products sold as dried fruit (eg, papaya and pineapples) are in fact candied fruit.

The specific nutrient content of various dried fruits reflect the nutrients in the original fruit. Fruits dried in the traditional manner will have almost the same nutrients as their fresh originals.

Fruits infused with sugar before drying will naturally be much sweeter than their fresh originals.

Drying, by definition, removes most of the water which concentrates the fruit's natural sugars. To obtain the same total sugar and energy, the amount of dried fruit you should eat should only be about 1/3 of the quantity of fresh fruit you would eat.

Prunes, dried dates, figs, apricots, peaches, apples and pears deliver energy when you are feeling tired and make great snacks ... provided they have been dried in the traditional manner without being infused in a sweetener.

But remember the water (two-thirds of a fruit on average) is gone, so watch carefully how much you eat.

26 - Minimising Unprocessed Animal Products

Much of the internet research I did on beating diabetes suggests that it would be best to give up unprocessed animal products entirely.

Because of the need for a balanced diet, ie one that delivers all nine essential amino acids on a daily basis, I'm not fully convinced. This is why I put fresh meat and fish in the eat-only-a-little category. I do ensure, of course, that the meat and fish I eat is ultra-lean.

On the plus side, animal products are major sources of protein in Western diets. On the minus side, however, animal products lack the fibre and carbohydrates everyone needs for good health.

They also contain significant amounts of fat and cholesterol. In fact, animal products are the only source of cholesterol in a diet, which is important to note because, being a diabetic, you most likely also have (or will have) cholesterol issues.

Reducing the amount of animal products you consume or eliminating them from your diet entirely can give you four main benefits ... (1) improved insulin sensitivity through the reduction of the fat inside your cells ... (2) reduced risk of cardio-vascular problems (that cause heart attacks, peripheral neuropathy, damaged eyes, etc) by the removal of cholesterol from your diet ... (3) reduction in or elimination of the harm animal proteins can cause your kidneys; and ... (4) reduced body weight.

Fats

For type 2 diabetics the prime problem, as I understand it, is that fat blocks the receptors in muscle cells and thus prevents insulin from doing its job of getting glucose into those cells. The purpose of the diet I use is to eliminate fats as much as possible in order to free up those receptors.

The problem with meat and fish for diabetics is that these foods deliver lots of fat. In addition, much of this fat is saturated fat.

Saturated fat is the 'bad' form of fat as, besides causing insulin insensitivity, it encourages the formation of cholesterol within your body.

About 50% of the fat in beef is saturated fat, as is about 30% of the fat in chicken. (Even if you discard the skin of a chicken and only eat the white flesh, you'll still get loads of fat ..... 23% of the calories in chicken come from fat!)

Between 15 to 30% of the fat in fish is saturated fat. All fish also have cholesterol. In fact, shrimp and lobster have more cholesterol than the same weight of steak.

Some people eat fish because it contains omega-3, a form of fat that blocks the formation of blood clots. However I noticed that some researchers now say that omega-3 (whether eaten in fish or as a supplement) does not offer any significant protection against cardiovascular disease, cancer, etc.

Most foods from plants (grains, beans, vegetables and fruits) contain very little fat. Indeed, with the exception of seeds, olives, avocados, nuts and some soy products, the percentage of calories you get from fat is much higher for meat and fish than it is for plant foods.

In animal products, the percentage of calories you get from fat ranges from 21% (white tuna) to 41% (lean loin of pork). Other examples include salmon caught in the Atlantic (40%), beef (37%), rainbow trout (35%), and skinless white of chicken (23%).

But when eating plants, the percentage of calories you get from fat is much less, ranging from a high of 11% for broccoli down to 3% for lentils and apples. Only 4% of the calories you get from eating navy beans and oranges are from fat, while for brown rice 7% of calories comes from fat.

My internet research suggests that a typical Western diet probably provides 80 to 100 grams of fat a day, if not more, plus at least 200mg a day of cholesterol. You can probably reduce this to about 60gm a day of fat by switching from beef to chicken or fish and by limiting added oils and keeping your portions quite small. But if you drop all animal products and added oils from your diet you can reduce your daily intake of fat to about 20gm and your cholesterol intake will be zero.

In my view, the best way to get the correct type and amount of fat is to eat lots of vegetables, fruit, beans and whole grains, and only a little lean meat or fish, and to avoid fried foods and other oily products and dairy products.

Cholesterol

Plants do not contain any cholesterol. Indeed meat and fish are the only sources of cholesterol in food.

A hundred grams of beef, for example, delivers 86mg of cholesterol. Chicken gives you 85mg per 100g, lean loin of pork 81mg, Atlantic salmon 71mg, rainbow trout 69mg, and white tuna 42mg.

If you don't eat any animal products, your diet will contain no cholesterol at all.

However, 75% or more of your cholesterol is manufactured by your body itself and it is encouraged to do so by saturated fat. Thus, by avoiding animal products you are also getting rid of a main impetus for the creation of cholesterol within your body.

Research shows that switching to a diet that contains only modest amounts of chicken and fish but eliminates meat from hoofed animals (beef, mutton, pork) reduces low-density lipoprotein (LDL) cholesterol, the so-called 'bad' cholesterol, by only 5%; but that eliminating all animal products reduces LDL by more than 20%. Thus, from the point of view of controlling cholesterol levels, it is four times better to give up animal products entirely.

Most of the damage diabetes does is to your arteries, which it clogs. This, in turn, leads to damage to your heart, eyes, kidneys and nerves. By getting your cholesterol under control, you should be able to avoid much of this damage.

Research suggests that if you can bring your cholesterol levels down you should experience relief from neuropathy, the painful nerve symptoms that arise as the nerves become damaged. In my experience this did not happen. I seem to have my cholesterol well under control, yet the damage to the nerves in my feet has not improved. However it has worsened only slightly.

Animal protein

The consensus of scientific opinion is that animal protein is harder on the kidneys than plant protein. I have seen statistics indicating that about 40% of diabetics have lost some kidney function.

Long-term studies indicate that the loss of kidney function varies with the amount of animal protein consumed, ie the more animal protein you consume then the more likely you are to suffer a loss of kidney function. For this reason, it is generally accepted that eating protein from plants is best.

Animal protein has other negative effects. It tends, for example, to cause calcium to pass through the kidneys and into the urine where it is lost but can, at the same time, cause stones in the urinary tract.

Obviously the smart thing would be to avoid animal protein or at least minimise your consumption of meat and fish.

Weight control

Traditional diets in places such as rural Africa and Asia are based on grains, vegetables and legumes. These foods are filling yet contain relatively few calories, so it's not surprising that the people who eat these foods tend to be slim.

In Europe and North Americas, the diet is based on meat and diary products which contain the calories stored in animal fat ... it can be no surprise that an obesity epidemic is sweeping the West.

It is obvious that if you switch from animal products to plants, you will lose weight as you will be taking in fewer calories. Indeed, statistics suggest that the switch can reduce your intake of calories by more than 50%.

However, to be sure, you may need to reduce your consumption of vegetable oil. Vegetable oils are lower in saturated fat than animal fats; this means they are better for you from the point of view of controlling cholesterol. However these 'good' fats do contain nine calories per gram (the same as animal fats) and are just as fattening as 'bad' animal fats.

Eating some fresh meat

If eliminating meat and fish from the diet has the four significant benefits indicated above, the question is: why don't I eliminate all meat from my diet and become a pure vegan?

There are two main reasons: (a) the risk of iron-deficiency, and (b) the need to maintain a balanced diet.

(a) **Risk of iron-deficiency** ... a lack of iron, a dietary mineral, in the diet can lead to anaemia. Anaemia is a serious problem that causes reduced physical performance and decreased cognitive functioning.

There are two kinds of iron in your diet. *Non-haem iron* is the form of iron found in plant foods, while *haem iron* is the kind you get from animal products.

Bioavailability refers to the extent to which a particular particle of food, such as a vitamin or mineral, is available, after being eaten, to the tissues it is intended to act upon.

The problem with a vegan diet is that the bioavailability of non-haem iron is much lower than that of haem iron. Thus persons who eat little or no meat are at an increased risk of iron-deficiency, which can develop into anaemia.

It is estimated that vegans may need almost twice as much dietary iron each day as non-vegans because of the lower intestinal absorption of non-haem iron.

Vitamin C, however, can double the absorption of non-haem iron. Some research indicates that it can quadruple absorption. Thus the usual recommendation is that vegans should eat plenty of citrus fruits, as they are rich in vitamin C, in order to improve the absorption of non-heme iron.

However, according to the Canadian researchers who discovered the ability of grapefruit to interact adversely with several medications (such as the statins used to control cholesterol levels), recent research suggest strongly that Seville oranges and limes have similar adverse effects. Research into the effects of other citrus fruits on commonly used medications is ongoing.

It seems to me that if some citrus fruits interfere with some medications, other citrus fruits are likely to have the same effect. Thus, as I use statins to control my cholesterol, I try to avoid all citrus fruits as far as possible. When I want to up my intake of vitamin C, I take a supplement. At the same time I continue to eat lean meat and fish in order to ensure that I get adequate amounts of haem iron.

(b) **Balanced diet** ... proteins, which are used to create and repair body tissues, are made up of small molecules called amino acids. There are at least 500 amino acids. However, only 20 are used for building proteins.

Most amino acids are created from other compounds within your body. However, your body cannot make nine of the amino acids needed to create proteins from its own resources. These are called essential amino acids as they have to be obtained in the food you eat.

Most meats contain all nine essential amino acids. Thus, if you eat some meat, you can be fairly sure that you are getting all the amino acids you need.

Plants are different. Certain plants contain particular amino acids but not others. If you can combine various vegetables and fruits properly you will get all the essential amino acids. This is known as a 'balanced' meal.

However, a fairly advanced knowledge of nutrition is needed to get this balance right. I do not have that knowledge.

The American Dietetic Association maintains that a plant-based diet will provide adequate protein without having to eat any particular combination of foods.

Nevertheless, most nutritionists are of the opinion that vegans need to ensure that, if they cannot get all the essential amino acids in one meal, they do get them all over the course of one day, ie that they eat a balanced daily diet.

For me, a diet containing moderate amounts of ultra-lean meat is much simpler.

27 - Minimising Vegetable Oils

The purpose of my diet is to eliminate fat, especially animal fats, from my food as far as possible in order to free up the receptors in my muscle cells. Our bodies however do need some fat.

What our bodies need, my research suggests, are tiny amounts of fat. Plants such as beans, grains and fruits contain trace amounts of oils, and these vegetable oils adequately fulfil our need for fats. What we do not need are the heavy amounts of oil we get with fried food and commercial products.

Vegetable oils have less saturated fat (which raises cholesterol levels) than animal fat, and for this reason are preferable to animal fats. However vegetable oils are just as fattening as animal fats. Both contain 9 calories per gram (while the calorific content of carbohydrate and protein is only 4 calories per gram) so we do need to restrict the amounts of vegetable oils we ingest.

There are two essential fats your body needs: alpha-linolenic acid and linoleic acid. *Alpha-linolenic acid* is the basic omega-3 fat the body uses to make the other fats it needs. Fish is a main source of omega-3 and related oils. The problem is that fish oil contains lots of saturated fats along with omega-3.

The good news is that these essential fats do not need to exceed 2 to 3 percent of your daily calorific intake and you can get all you need from plant foods. The trace amounts of fats in beans, vegetables and fruit are relatively rich in these essential fats. Nuts, seeds and soy products contain even larger amounts.

However, the oil contents of several plant foods, including most nuts, some soy products, seeds, avocados, and olives, are naturally high. I try to avoid these or at least minimise their consumption.

Olive oil, for example, is made by pulping olives. The resulting liquid is pure fat. Gram for gram, it has the same calories (9) as other fats and oils. About 13% of it is saturated fat which worsens insulin resistance and increases cholesterol.

As well as avoiding animal oils (including fish oils) you need to ensure that vegetable oils do not exceed 2 to 3 percent of your daily calorific intake. It would be silly, once you have regained some insulin sensitivity by avoiding animal fats, to gum up your muscle cells again with vegetable fat.

Vegetable oils in our diets

As far as I can figure it out there are four main sources of vegetable oils in our diets: (a) snack foods; (b) dressings and spreads; (c) packaged products; and (d) cooking.

Nowadays a vast array of snacks is available in every supermarket, corner store and chipper. These include all sorts of confectionary (sweets, chocolates and 'energy' bars) as well as chips (French fries), potato crisps (chips), onion rings, and other fried snacks.

Lots of vegetable oils are added to dressings and margarines to improve texture and 'spreadability', while many of the packaged sauces and foods you can buy contain oil as an ingredient.

Cooking can be a prime source of added oils. Many recipes require individual ingredients (eg, onions, garlic or chunks of flesh) to be pan-fried, sautéed or deep-fried in oil ... to 'lock-in flavours' before the ingredients are brought together in the final dish.

Reducing oils

Avoiding all this gunge is surprisingly easy. For a start, you don't really need snacks ... they're just a habit. Eat a piece of fruit or other permissible food instead.

Don't smear your bread with butter, margarine or other spreads. Wholemeal breads come in a variety of textures and flavours and you'll be surprised how quickly you'll learn to appreciate these once you are no longer submerging them in gunge.

You can avoid oil laden dressings by using lemon juice, balsamic vinegar or fat-free dressings on your salads. And you can reduce the oil contained in the packaged sauces and other food products you buy by getting used to reading the labels ... only go for products in which less than 10% of the calories come from fat or which only have 2 (or at most 3) grams of fat per serving.

Minimising the amount of oil you use to cook is also fairly easy and straightforward. Avoid the deep-fryer which is totally unnecessary, and grill rather than fry. When you do have to fry or sauté, use a non-stick pan to minimise the need for oil and, rather than pouring oil into the pan for frying, use a cooking-spray to coat ingredients in oil instead.

I read somewhere that you can use water instead of oil for frying or sautéing which, if it worked, would be a great way to eliminate added oil from your cooking. I've tried it. It sorta worked but not very well. But you might be luckier than me.

You should of course steam or boil your vegetables.

The best way to get the correct type and amount of fat is to eat lots of vegetables, fruit, beans and whole grains and avoid fried foods, oily food products and dairy products, and only eat a little lean meat or fish.

By switching to a plant-focused diet and eliminating fats as much as possible, you will:

(1) increase your insulin sensitivity ... because fat is no longer blocking your cell receptors

(2) lose weight (which in turn helps your insulin sensitivity) ... because (a) fat (the main source of unwanted calories) has been reduced dramatically ... (b) you are getting more fibre (which turns off your appetite a bit sooner; each 14gms of fibre cuts about 10% off your calorie intake) ... and (c) your after-meal calorie burn is boosted a bit.

(3) improve your cholesterol levels, as you are taking in very little cholesterol

(4) reverse symptoms of nerve damage provided you combine your change of diet with a programme of vigorous exercise.

28 - Eggs a No-No ... along with the fry-up

It wasn't until I gave up eggs, fried foods and dairy products that my diet began to have a positive effect on my health.

Eggs are out

I feel that avoiding eggs is crucial to beating my diabetes ... it's not hard to understand why when you consider what they are made of.

An egg consists of a yellow yoke surrounded by 'white'. The yoke is essentially pure fat ... 5 grams of fat and over 200mg of cholesterol in a normal-sized hen's egg. That's as much cholesterol as you'll find in a large 8oz steak.

The egg white is basically pure animal protein, which is not surprising as a chick has to be formed from just the contents inside the shell. This makes eggs an excellent source of protein for humans, albeit animal protein which is hard on the kidneys and comes with a massive dose of animal fat.

Fat and protein ... that's what you get from eggs. Eggs do not contain any complex carbohydrates or dietary fibre. The lack of carbohydrate means that eggs do not appear on the glycemic index.

As well as being great sources of protein, eggs also deliver plenty of vitamins and dietary minerals, including vitamins B7 (biotin), B12 and D, and iron, all of which are important for health and well-being.

Eggs therefore would appear to be a pretty necessary part of the human diet, as least as far as micro-nutrients are concerned. The short answer is 'yes but ...'

The problem is the vast quantities of animal fat (and cholesterol) you have to ingest just to get those micro-nutrients, which is why I have cut eggs out of my diet.

However, in doing so, I was eliminating an important source of some very necessary vitamins and minerals from my diet. This is why, if you follow my example, you must ... absolutely must ... take dietary supplements to make up for any shortfalls.

So is the fry-up

Fried eggs, rashers of bacon, sausages, black and white puddings, fried bread, grilled tomatoes and mushrooms, baked beans, and pan-fried potato cakes ... the ingredients of the traditional breakfast or evening fry-up ... will be no help at all in beating your diabetes.

You have to cut this culinary delight out completely, with the possible exception of the grilled tomatoes and mushrooms, and baked beans.

Here's why ... the dish is loaded with fat, cholesterol and salt.

Eggs ... frying adds substantially to the 50% fat eggs already contain.

Bacon ... cured pork contains around 38% protein. A rasher is also a good source of niacin, phosphorus and selenium. However it delivers saturated fat, cholesterol and sodium in the sort of doses that will prevent you beating your diabetes.

A 100g of back bacon (about two rashers) will contain 40g of fat, of which 13g will be saturated, and 110mg of cholesterol. Indeed 68% of its calories will come from fat.

If you insist on eating bacon, choose low-salt back bacon (not streaky), trim off all visible fat and grill it rather than fry it.

In my view, it is better to give rashers up entirely so that your taste buds change and you get used to a low fat diet of natural (unprocessed) foods.

Sausages ... no doubt pork sausages are a good source of protein. However they also contain about 28% fat, including 9% saturated fat and some trans fats, as well as 84mg of cholesterol per 100g. Fat accounts for 75% of the calories in pork sausages.

Sausages also contain high levels of salt, around 750mg per 100g, both as a flavour enhancer and as a preservative. Sausages are out ... no exceptions.

Black and white puddings ... are high in saturated fat (with a total fat content of about 15%) and salt.

Fried bread ... even the purest of wholemeal will, after frying, contain at least 15% fat.

So, if you are really serious about beating your diabetes, you must forget about the traditional fried breakfast.

Try beans on wholemeal toast with grilled tomato and mushroom on the side ... much healthier and equally delicious.

Personally, I have porridge (oatmeal) instead.

29 - No-No to Dairy Products

There are good reasons for eliminating dairy products ... milk, cream, yoghurt, cheese, butter and so on ... from a diet designed to beat type 2 diabetes.

Dairy products provide you with lots of ... fat ... cholesterol ... sugar ... and animal protein.

Fat

All dairy products are made from milk and most of them are high in fat.

There are four types of milk. (a) Whole (full-fat) milk contains about 3.25% fat by weight, ie 100g (less than half a glass) will contain over 3 grams of fat. (b) Reduced-fat milk contains 2% fat by weight and (c) low-fat milk just 1%. (d) Skim (non-fat) milk only contains trace amounts of fat.

Calories from fat ... the thing about milk is that it is mostly water. This makes measuring the amount of fat (or other ingredients) by weight in milk meaningless.

In my internet research I discovered that nutritionists prefer to measure the fat in liquids (and in other foods) by measuring the calories you get from fat as a percentage of the total calories you get from a particular food.

Here's the calories you get from fat in cow's milk ... whole milk, about 49% ... reduced (2%) milk, about 35% ... low-fat (1%) milk, about 20% of calories from fat.

For skim milk, of course, you should get no calories from fat. But in fact it's impossible to make the milk entirely fat free but you do get less than 5% of calories from fat with skim milk.

The percentage of calories that come from fat is unaffected by the water content of the milk. As you can see, even low-fat milk contains a lot of fat.

Many other dairy products are loaded with fat. If you eat yoghurt, about 47% of calories come from fat. With cheese, up to 70% of calories come from fat depending on the type of cheese (and I don't recommend fat-free cheese ... it tastes like sanitised rubber ... so forget about cheese).

As for sour cream ... almost 90% of calories come from fat ... 87% for reduced-fat version!

Butter is hardly any better. Commercial butter consists of up to 82% fat, 16% or so water, and up to 2% curd, ie milk solids other than fat. This butter may also contain up to 2% salt, another no-no if you have blood pressure problems (which are twice as common in diabetics as non-diabetics).

The best plan is to give up all dairy products because, with the exception of skim milk or other dairy products from which fat has been removed, dairy-based foodstuffs will block the receptors in your muscle cells and make it very difficult to beat your diabetes.

Cholesterol

Most of the fat in milk and dairy products is saturated, the kind that raises cholesterol levels and ups your insulin resistance. Indeed, all full-fat dairy products contain copious amounts of cholesterol.

If you are trying to control your cholesterol the first thing you have to do is eliminate (or at least severely restrict) the cholesterol you ingest in your food. Doing this would be impossible if you drink or eat dairy products, even if you limit yourself to the 'low-fat' kinds.

For instance, 100g of full-fat sour cream contains 52mg of cholesterol. Even fat-free sour cream has 9mg of cholesterol in 100g, almost as much as whole cows milk (10mg per 100g, ie, only about 1/3rd of a cup). A 100g of plain yoghurt made from whole milk will deliver 13mg of cholesterol.

Besides 'fat-free' sour cream, other non-fat dairy products contain some cholesterol. Skim milk has about 2mg per 100g, as does plain yoghurt made from the same kind of milk.

As you have type 2 diabetes there is an 85% chance that you also have cholesterol issues. When you consider the dire consequences of clogged arteries, the need to give up dairy products becomes obvious.

Sugar

The kind of sugar you get in milk is lactose, which is a combination of glucose and galactose, two simple sugars. This dairy sugar occurs in the milk of mammals ... about 5% by weight in cow's milk and up to 8% in human milk ... and is the main nutrient in skim milk after the fat has been taken out.

Most dairy products contain carbohydrates in the form of lactose. Even high-fat cheeses and heavy creams contain a little. Only one dairy product ... butter ... is totally sugar free.

Lactose is broken down in the intestinal tract by an enzyme called lactase so that its two simple sugars can be absorbed and used for energy. When mammals are being weaned they usually stop drinking milk regularly and production of the enzyme decreases gradually as they grow older.

However, due to a genetic mutation, many people with ancestry in Europe, West Asia, India and parts of East Africa continue to tolerate lactase and can continue to drink milk into adulthood. Other people, who do not have the modified gene, suffer from wind, cramps and diarrhoea when they drink milk. This is known as *lactose intolerance*.

Lactose intolerance affects up to 30% of adults of European descent and more than 70% of adults from parts of Africa, East and South-east Asia and the Pacific islands.

The problem with being lactose tolerant is that you, as a type 2 diabetic, do not need to take in more sugar than absolutely necessary and drinking animal milk and dairy products certainly will not help you minimise your intake.

All cows' milk, fat-free or not, contains about 5% sugar by weight. However the percentage of calories derived from carbohydrates runs from just under 30% for whole milk to 54% for skim milk. The figures for plain yoghurt are more or less the same.

Sour cream is the killer ... when made from whole milk it contains 8% carbohydrates but less than 6% of the calories come from carbohydrates. However, fat-free sour cream contains 16% carbohydrates which deliver 83% of its calories.

Casein, the milk protein

Milk contains all the essential amino acids. The major protein in cows' milk is casein (80%), the milk protein. Casein also makes up 20 to 45% of the proteins found in human milk.

Casein has a wide variety of uses. It is a major component in cheese-making. It is also used as a food additive in, for example, non-dairy creamers and soy cheeses. In addition, casein is processed into food supplements, such as calcium caseinate, which are used to enrich foodstuffs with amino-acids, improve other nutritional features, enhance their taste and smell, and increase their shelf life. To avoid casein in your diet must read food labels closely ... this is absolutely necessary.

Cheese consists of proteins and fat from milk. It is made by coagulating the casein in the milk. This is usually done by acidifying the milk and then adding rennet (which contains the required enzyme). The solids (up to 70% fat) that result are taken out of the liquid and pressed into shape.

All the fat in cheese certainly has to be avoided by type 2 diabetics. But it's not just the fat and lactose in dairy products that can be damaging. It's the dairy protein itself.

All animal protein, including dairy protein, accelerates the gradual loss of kidney function that can occur with diabetes, while protein obtained from plants does not have this effect. As far as I can tell, this is received opinion among medical scientists and nutritionists.

Casein has, in addition, been linked to problems, such as migraines, rheumatoid arthritis, and prostrate and ovarian cancers, which do not seem to occur with other animal proteins. People who suffer from migraines and persons who have rheumatoid arthritis often experience improvements when they avoid milk and other dairy products. According to the reports I have read the problem for these people seems to be the proteins, not the lactose or fat, in dairy products.

By experimenting on animals, researchers have shown that there is a consistent correlation between the growth of cancers and the amount of casein in a diet. Indeed, statistics show that men who drink milk have a significantly higher risk of prostate cancer than non-milk drinkers. In addition, some studies show that women who drink milk have a higher risk of ovarian cancer than non-drinkers. But other studies show no heightened risk.

Micro-nutrients

Milk is a good source of vitamins D, B2 (riboflavin) and B12, and of calcium and phosphorus, as well as some selenium. Many of these vitamins and minerals, along with magnesium and potassium, are also found in significant quantities in cheeses, yoghurts and sour creams. It seems a pity to have to give up dairy products.

And so it is. But the benefits you get from these micro-nutrients are far outweighed by the damage fat, sugar and casein and other animal proteins in milk and dairy products can cause you, especially as you are a type 2 diabetic. You just have to take supplements instead, to replace those vital micro-nutrients.

Once of the reasons given for drinking milk regularly is the calcium it contains, as you need constant intakes of calcium to avoid osteoporosis in old age. That's true. However, you get plenty of calcium from green leafy vegetables (such as spinach, kale or broccoli) and beans and peas, as well as from very cheap calcium supplements that also contain the vitamin D needed to absorb the calcium.

Another reason to stop consuming dairy products is that they are usually low in iron and tend to inhibit its absorption from the digestive tract.

Substitutes for dairy products

There are plenty of substitutes for dairy products. Just look around your local supermarket. You have, however, to be careful that they do not contain any casein which is often sneaked in as an additive or food supplement.

Substitutes for animal milk include soy milk, oat milk, rice milk and almond milk, and a host of other milks made from plants. Soy milk is undoubtedly the most popular worldwide. After soy, oat milk is the best-selling plant-milk in Europe, while rice and almond are the most common in the USA. You can also get milk made from hazelnuts and coconuts as well as from peas and lupins, though I have yet to try the last two.

Plant-based milks, like animal milks, can be low-fat and calcium-fortified and can come in various flavours. There are, however, three things you should beware of: added casein, sugar and fat.

Casein and its caseinate derivatives may sometimes be added to plant milks and you need to check labels carefully. You also need to check the sugar content (as sugar may be added to enhance taste) and fat. And any milk should contain less than 3% fat and only 10% of its energy should come from fat.

You should be equally cautious when choosing other substitutes for dairy products. Vegan ice cream, for example, may be delicious because it has added sugar. Be especially cautious of vegetarian products ... many of them contain dairy proteins and/or egg whites. You should choose the vegan versions and the ones that are lowest in fat.

Personally I use soy milk to drink, put in my coffee for a latte, and for my porridge. I find it delicious and had no problem in switching over from cows milk. Then, once I began researching the matter, I discovered that soy milk does not contain the high doses of saturated fats found in animal-based milk. I also found some research that suggests that soy may be able to lower cholesterol levels.

As regards other dairy-based products, I have dropped these entirely. I don't eat any sour cream, cheese or butter. I occasionally eat some non-dairy yoghurt which I enjoy. I regret not being able to eat cheese but not too intensely.

I had thought that I would really miss butter (I strongly dislike margarines) and was surprised to find that this was not so. In fact, strange to say, I rather enjoy dry bread or toast, especially if it has some raisins or other small bits of fruit in it.

30 - More Foods to Avoid

To beat your diabetes you need to control the fat and sugar in your diet. In my view, controlling the fat is probably the more important of the two ... after all, it is the fat that is blocking the receptors in your muscle cells.

That's not to say, of course, that you can ignore the sugar in what you eat.

You also need to ensure that your diet is low in salt but high in fibre, and that the food you eat is low on the glycemic index. The easiest way to do all this is to list the foods that you cannot eat, rather than list the foods you should eat.

Once you have the no-no list in place, you can eat everything else, albeit some things (eg, fresh fish and lean meat) only in moderation.

The criteria I use for deciding whether a food should go on the no-no list are very simple ... fat ... sugar ... salt ... fibre ... and GI ranking. Nothing could be simpler provided you can find the data you need.

Eggs and dairy products are at the top of my no-no list. Here are some more foods I avoid.

Processed meats

The benefits and hazards of processed foods have been discussed in chapter 11. These foods are, in the main, less susceptible to spoilage than fresh foods and have more consistent (and often much improved) nutritional values. They are also convenient and cheap.

However, processed foods can contain excessive amounts of fats (including trans-fats), sugar and salt. In addition they may contain harmful additives and preservatives.

It's hard to avoid eating some processed foods. But, as a type 2 diabetic, you need to be especially wary of processed meats. These can be divided into six categories according to the UN's FAO (Food & Agricultural Organisation):

[1] Fresh-processed meat products ... such as hamburgers, fresh sausages, kebabs, and chicken nuggets ... are made by pulverising raw muscle-meat and mixing in varying quantities of animal fat and loads of salt. Already full of fat and salt, these have to be fried before they are eaten, adding lots more fat.

[2] Cured meats ... such as cured-raw ham and beef, cured-cooked beef, ham and bacon ... are made from whole pieces of muscle-meat. They are first cured using a mixture of common salt (99.5%) and sodium nitrite (0.5%). Cured-raw meats are then allowed to ferment or ripen in a climate-controlled environment and are eaten uncooked, while cured-cooked meats are treated with heat after curing.

[3] Raw-cooked meat products ... such as frankfurters, mortadella, and meat loaf ... are made by pulverising muscle meats, fat and non-meat ingredients and mixing them together. The viscous mix is formed into sausage or other shapes and then treated with heat which coagulates the protein.

[4] Pre-cooked products ... such as black pudding (blood sausage), liver pate and corned beef in cans ... are made from mixtures of muscle trimmings, fatty tissues, head meat, animal feet, animal skin, blood, liver and other edible by-products of butchering. The raw meat materials are first pre-cooked and then ground or chopped and mixed together. They are then cooked for a second time.

[5] Raw-fermented sausages ... such as salami and related products ... consist of mixtures of lean meats and fatty tissues combined in casings with salt, nitrite (a curing agent), sugar, spices and non-meat ingredients. They are not heat treated and their flavours depend on the fermentation process and length of the ripening period. They are eaten raw.

[6] Dried meats ... such as beef jerky and African biltong ... consist of lean meat that has been dried naturally. The meat is cut into strips or flat pieces with a uniform shape so that they dry gradually at an equal rate. Many of the nutritional properties of meat, especially the protein, are not affected by drying and its shelf-life is much longer than fresh meat.

As you can see, processed meat products (except for dried meats) are mixtures of lean meats, fatty meats, and non-meat ingredients. Many contain salts and nitrites, and sugars. Some have to be fried either in the pan or a deep-fat fryer before being eaten. They certainly would not help you beat your type 2 diabetes and have a prominent position on my no-no list.

All are therefore off the menu with a possible exception of naturally-dried meats (eg, beef jerky) provided salt has not been added during the drying process.

The only other (occasional) exception is boiled ham (a cured meat), provided it is unglazed. I use an old trick to get rid of the salt ... soaking the ham in plain water overnight (for up to 24 hours) and discarding the water before cooking. You'll see the salt floating away. You then hard-boil the ham for about 10 minutes before changing the water again. After that you boil the ham in the usual way until it is cooked. The soaking trick seems to get rid of most of the salt used to cure the pork.

Nuts

Nuts are rich in energy and protein, packed with antioxidants, vitamins, minerals and omega-3 fatty acids. They are, without a doubt, storehouses of high quality nutrients and you should eat a handful a day ... unless you are a type 2 diabetic.

Nuts are especially rich in fats ... too rich for type 2 diabetics. Macadamias and pecan nuts have the highest fat content, with more than 70g per 100g. Even the least caloric, cashews and pistachios, contain more than 40g of fat in a 100g. And, on average, 60% of the calories in nuts come from fats. If you have managed to improve your insulin sensitivity by unblocking the receptors in your muscle cells, the fats you get from eating a few nuts will quickly block them up again.

The fats in nuts are mostly unsaturated and are therefore beneficial in preventing heart disease and lowering LDL cholesterol. However, some nuts such as Brazil nuts, macadamias, cashews and pine nuts also contain large amounts of saturated fats.

Properly conducted research indicates that certain nuts, such as almonds and walnuts, can actually lower cholesterol. Even though they are as high in fat as other nuts, they have the (unexplained) ability to reduce cholesterol levels. Measurable reductions in cholesterol when 3 ounces (a large handful) a day are eaten for 4 weeks have been recorded.

Thus for most people, nuts are a very healthy food. However their fat content rules them out for diabetics ... their fattiness would make weight difficult to control and most likely to worsen insulin insensitivity ... which is why they are on my no-no list.

Grains

Grain products range from breakfast food through the carbohydrates we eat for dinner to a vast range of baked products. As a general rule, you can eat all you want (within reason) of foods based on whole grains but should be very cautious of foods made using refined grains.

Dinner grains

I call grains such as rice and pasta, which you eat with a main course, *dinner grains*.

The no-noes are the grains which have had their bran and germ removed. These refined grains include white rice, pearl or pearled barley, noodles made from refined grains (read the labels), leavened pasta, well-cooked pasta and pasta made with eggs.

The best dinner grains for type 2 diabetics are unrefined grains: brown rice, barley (great in soup, a stew, as a side dish, or mixed with rice), rye berries, savoury semolina, bulgur wheat (in soup, casseroles or as a side dish), couscous, noodles made from whole grains and unleavened wholemeal pasta cooked al-dente.

Sometimes I feel that all pasta should be on the no-no list. To cook it just enough to make it digestible but not enough to cause its GI to go up requires precision timing.

Breakfast cereals

Personally I prefer to set myself up for the day with a big bowl of porridge made from whole oats to which I add extra oat bran, a good bit of wheat bran, half a cup of blueberries and other berries, and a small banana, as well as a sprinkling of cinnamon powder. I use soy milk rather than cow's milk.

Despite the fruit, two hours after eating this high carbohydrate meal, my glucose levels are about 6mmol per litre, the middle of my target range. I urge you to follow suit and eat a low-GI breakfast.

However, 'quick' or 'instant' oatmeal to which you just add boiling water to make your porridge is a no-no. A properly nutritious porridge is made from oatmeal that you have to simmer in water (preferably overnight) or cook in a micro-wave oven.

Whatever breakfast cereal you use, make sure it is made from whole-grains and does not have lots of added sugar. If you prefer a cold cereal, Wheetabix and All Bran should be OK. But the cereals designed to appeal to children, such as Coco Pops and Clusters, are definite no-noes ... just check the ingredients and nutritional values ... they are jammed full of sugar.

Commercial Muesli is also a no-no ... unless you can find one that is sugar-free, untoasted and not too full of nuts. You can always make up your own version of Muesli by combining whole grains from different cereals and adding fresh fruit. Leave out the nuts and eat it with soy milk.

Baked products
When choosing what bread, pastries and cakes to buy, check the contents for protein, fat, sugar, salt, fibre, and GI ranking. Fat should be limited to 3% by weight and energy from fat should not exceed 10%. Needless to say, baked products should also be low in sugar and salt, high in fibre, and have a low GI ranking.

While many types of bread meet these criteria, few pastries and almost no cakes can be eaten by type 2 diabetics.

Bread
Among breads, the major no-no is white bread, ie bread made from refined flour, and brown bread, ie white bread that has been coloured.

Other breads you should treat with extreme caution include wheat germ bread which is ordinary white bread with some added wheat germ for flavouring, granary bread which is basically white or brown flour mixed with flaked wheat grains, and whole-grain bread which is white bread to which whole grains have been added ... you'll recognize it from the small print on the label which will read something like: '60% whole-grain bread.'

Why settle for less than 100% whole grain bread when it is readily available, and just as nutritious as (and tastier than) white bread with extra bits? As far as I can judge, refining flour is much profitable than selling wholegrain flour because the bran and germ that have been removed (semolina) to make refined grains can be used in other products (eg, couscous) and have a market value.

Other no-noes include quick-breads, eg Irish soda bread, unless these have been made from wholemeal flour, and breads in which excessive amounts of salt has been used as an improver. You need to check the salt content on the label.

No-noes also include fried bread, such as Indian puri, because of the fat. Where shortening (such as butter, lard, oils or egg fat) has been used you should check the label to ensure that the fat content is not more than 3% by weight ... if it's more than 3%, treat the bread as a no-no.

Wholemeal bread usually has a good GI ranking. Some bread is now marked 'Low GI' ... which I assume means it is wholemeal and that bread which is not marked as low GI is likely to have a high GI.

The good breads you can eat are wholemeal breads, rye breads such as pumpernickel, crisp breads made from rye flour, unleavened flatbreads (provided they do not contain too much salt), and Indian roti and chapatti (unleavened whole-wheat Indian breads). There breads can be even better if they have been fortified with additional vitamins and dietary minerals.

Pastries
Most pastries, as you will have noticed in the chapter on grains, are full of fat in the form of shortenings and glazes. Many are also full of sugar, though this is more likely due to the fillings and non-pastry ingredients.

The real no-noes include Danish pastries and croissant, brioche, mille-feuille, profiteroles and éclairs, and any other pastries that have additional fat or sugar in their make-up or their fillings.

The flaky texture of Danish pastries and croissants comes from repeatedly rolling out the yeast-leavened dough, spreading it with butter and folding it over. This laminating technique adds butter (ie, fat) by the bucketful. Danish pastries, in addition, are usually sodden with sweetened syrup.

Brioche is not really a pastry. It's highly enriched bread loaded with egg and butter which gives it a tender sweet crumb (interior) but makes it is totally unsuitable for beating your diabetes.

Mille-feuille, sometimes called custard or vanilla slice, is traditionally made with three layers of puff pastry and two layers of pastry cream (or whipped cream or jam) in between. The top may be dusted with sugar, cocoa or pulverized roast almonds, or glazed with icing or fondant (a creamy confection made from sugar or water).

While the topping makes mille-feuille an absolute no-no, the layers of pastry cream reinforce its no-no status drastically.

Indeed, to beat your diabetes, you need to avoid pastry products containing pastry cream, aka confectioner's custard. This is made from egg and flour using sweetened milk (often flavoured with vanilla). The purpose of the flour is to prevent the egg from curdling. Pastry cream is used as a filling in pastries, tarts, flans and cakes, and the egg and sweetened milk means that it will have an adverse effect on your blood glucose levels. You can only avoid it by reading labels attentively.

Profiteroles, cream puffs, choux a la creme, eclairs and so on are all variations on a theme ... choux pastry balls or tubes filled with whipped cream, pastry cream or ice cream, often garnished with chocolate or caramel sauce or given a good dusting of powdered sugar. It's a pity, sometimes, to be a diabetic.

So what pastries can you eat? Not many. You can probably eat fruit pies made with simple pasty provided no sugar has been added to the fruit. I enjoy a homemade fresh fruit pie made with simple unsweetened puff pastry covered in unsweetened soy-based custard once a week. But that's about it.

Cakes

Every cake is a no-no ... due to the oodles of fat and sugar, whether in the cakes themselves or their decorative coverings. There are no exceptions ... none at all, if you truly want to beat your diabetes.

No-no vegetables

Vegetables are a fundamental part of my diet for beating my diabetes, and there are only two vegetables I avoid: olives and avocados ... due to the fat they contain ... as well as tinned vegetables with added sugar.

Most vegetables contain less than 1% fat by weight. However, olives have a fat content that can range from 15% to as high as 35%, while avocados contain about 15% fat.

But the type of fat they contain is considered benign (provided you are not diabetic) and these two vegetables also contain other healthful substances and may be effective in preventing certain diseases as mentioned in the chapter on vegetables. My view, nevertheless, is that the heavy fat content more than negates these positive attributes and I can always find other sources of any nutrients I am missing.

Tinned vegetables with added sugar are another no-no. Why manufacturers have to add sugar I don't know. But sometimes they do, and you need to read the labels closely. Look out for 'Sugar Free' and 'No Added Sugar' tags on the tin and read the small print.

Potatoes I am wary of. They have a relatively high GI compared to most other vegetables, which is why I eat yams or sweet-potatoes instead as often as possible. Boiled potatoes are OK, once in a while, but I avoid oil-cooked spuds such as chips (French fries) and roast potatoes, as well as crisps (chips in America).

Indeed, I eschew all fried vegetables except, occasionally, I will eat stir-fried vegetables that have been flash fried and then drained thoroughly using oil-absorbent paper.

No-no fruits
Fruit is also a significant part of my diet. However many kinds of fruit are more sugar heavy than vegetables and so need to be treated with a greater degree of caution by diabetics. In addition, a few also contain high levels of fat, albeit vegetable fats. Here are my no-no fruits:

Crystallised fruits ... aka candied or glacé fruit ... are small pieces of fruit or peal that have been preserved using sugar. The fruit is drenched with sugar syrup, and once it has become saturated the sugar prevents the micro-organisms that spoil fruit from growing.

Crystallised fruits can include dates, cherries, pineapple, ginger and chestnuts (marron glacé), as well as orange and lemon peel.

Sugar-infused dried fruit ... fruit soaked in sugar syrup prior to drying ... will send your glucose levels soaring and is therefore a total no-no ... as are dried papaya and pineapple which are actually crystallised (candied) fruit.

You can eat traditional sun/hot-air dried fruit but only about one-third of what you would eat of the fresh fruit equivalent.

Tinned (canned) fruits with added sugar ... are my next no-no. Why canners have to add sugar to fruit I cannot fathom ... there are plenty of natural sugars in fruit so the extra sugar is totally unnecessary. You need to read the labels closely.

Fruit juices with added sugar... are also a no-no. For example, sugar is often added to juices such as apple and orange for no good reason in my view. Read the labels and stick to unsweetened juices.

Cranberry juice ... is very tart and so may justifiably be sweetened. But that's no good for a diabetic. You can, however, find unsweetened cranberry juice and I must admit that I enjoy its tartness ... if you persist you too will probably come to like the unadulterated taste of this super-juice.

Fruits high in sugar in their natural state ... are also no-noes. Fresh ripe dates contain about 60% sugar by weight (and not much less if they are dried dates), though their GI numbers are reasonable. Figs contain somewhat less sugar, 48% by weight, and grapes, the next sweetest, about 15%.

I avoid dates and figs entirely and only very occasionally nibble on a very small bunch of grapes.

Fruits high in fat ... include coconut and açaí. Coconut contains a whopping 33.5g of fat per 100g, of which 90% is saturated. And that wondrous cure-all açaí has almost the same total amount of fat ... 32.5%. For a diabetic, both must be on the no-no list.

Grapefruit ... is a definite no-no. More than 85 different drugs ... many of which are prescribed for common medical conditions such as elevated cholesterol levels ... may interact with grapefruit according to the *Canadian Medical Association Journal*.

All the drugs affected by grapefruit have low bio-availability because an enzyme in the liver (CYP3A4) normally inactivates these drugs, so much higher doses than would be otherwise necessary must be taken. What the grapefruit does is inhibit the enzyme CYP3A4 from doing its job.

This effect is evident even if the grapefruit is eaten many hours before taking the medicine. Properly conducted clinical trials show that a patient on simvastatin, a statin, who drinks a glass of grapefruit juice every day for three days will experience at least a three-fold rise in the concentration of the drug in his or her system compared to another patient who drinks water instead of grapefruit juice.

The serious side-effects you can get from eating grapefruit or drinking the juice while on these drugs include acute kidney failure, respiratory failure and gastro-intestinal bleeding especially as (being a diabetic) your immune system is compromised.

That is why I never touch grapefruit.

The reason grapefruit acts this way is due to the furanocoumarins it contains. These are chemical compounds produced by a variety of plants. Many furanocoumarins are toxic and their purpose is to defend the plants from insect or animal predators; eg, the juice of the wild parsnip will give you dermatitis. Two particular furanocoumarins, bergamottin and dihydroxybergamottin, contained in grapefruit affect the metabolism of 85 drugs.

Other citrus fruit ... the two furanocoumarins that produce the grapefruit juice effect are present in other citrus fruits such as limes and Seville oranges. As to whether these citrus fruits also affect the metabolism of vital drugs, research is ongoing. But as they are the same furanocoumarins I'd prefer not to wait for the official results ... I avoid all other citrus fruits as far as possible.

Commercially made fruit products ... such as jams, desserts, pies and crumbles ... usually contain oodles of sugar. In addition, due to the liberal use of shortenings and glazes, the pastry cases of pies and crumbles are full of fat.

Thus, I avoid eating these fruit products.

The only exception I make is to occasionally use a thin smear of jam which has been made without adding sugar on toast.

I also eat home-made fruit pies made with home-made pastry that has been made without any added sugar. Needless to say, no sugar has been added to the fruit also. I enjoy this indulgence no more than once a week when I top the pie with a soy-based custard.

Other fruits ... though they are not no-noes, you need to exercise restraint when eating peaches and nectarines, plums, prunes, cranberries, strawberries, pomegranates, banana, melon, kiwifruit, as they are higher in sugar than other fruits.

Water melon and pineapple should also be eaten cautiously as they have much higher GIs than other fruits, ie their sugars will be released quickly into the bloodstream.

Fried foods

Foods cooked by frying, especially deep-frying, are total no-noes. The only (occasional) exceptions are foods that are pan-fried quickly using a minimum of oil.

Fats and oils

Absolute no-noes include all animal fats and oils such as butter, suet and dripping. I also exclude margarine from my diet because, even though they are made from plant rather than animal fats, most margarine consists of more than 80% fat!

While I don't treat it as an absolute no-no, I do use only very tiny amounts of olive oil. This is because even though 72% by weight consists of healthful monounsaturated fats and olive oil contains a wide range of antioxidants not found in other oils, it is still 100% an oil and therefore likely to block the receptors in my muscle cells ... not all healthful foods are healthful for diabetics!

Though they are healthier than animal fats, I also minimise the plant oils ... corn oil, sunflower oil, soy oil, safflower and rapeseed oil ... in my diet as these are fats (like all other fats) that can clog my muscle receptors.

Sauces, dressings and condiments

Many sauces and condiments, such as redcurrant sauce and redcurrant jelly, are made by first boiling the berries with sugar ... so obviously these are no-noes due to their sugar content. Dressings, such as salad dressing and mayonnaise, are high in fat and are therefore no-noes also.

Commercial vinaigrettes should also be no-noes but I find that a light sprinkling on my salads does no harm. It is possible to make fat-free vinaigrette by substituting a mixture of water, low-sodium vegetarian broth powder and cornstarch for the oil in traditional vinaigrette and I have done so with success. But I don't do so very often out of sheer laziness.

You should be able to spice your food up with herbs and spices without any problem. In addition, sauces such as Tabasco and Worcestershire sauce as well as other similar sauces should also be OK ... however you need to check the labels carefully for their fat, sugar and salt content. You also need to check the labels before using condiments such as pickles and chutneys.

Jams, preserves and spreads

Jams and marmalades (including low-sugar versions), peanut butter, and fish and meat pastes are all in the no-no category. However there are some commercial jams that are made without sugar so an occasional smear of these on toast may be OK, if you can find them in your local shop.

Honey is basically all sugar so, despite any miraculous ingredients it may or may not contain (depending on your gullibility), it is a total no-no.

But occasionally using Marmite and Bovril as a spread should be OK, though you should check the labels.

Artificial sweeteners

Though many artificial sweeteners are not no-noes because they contain excessive sugar or fat, I never use non-sugar sweeteners at all for one simple reason ... to retrain my taste-buds.

All the foods we like are acquired tastes, with the sole exception of mother's milk. This is obvious if you consider the length of time and repetitive effort it takes to wean a child. Remember your first taste of certain vegetables or your first glass of beer? Of course we can acquire some tastes quickly, especially when they are variations on tastes with which we are already familiar.

My contention is that the tastes we have acquired can be 'de-acquired', ie if we don't experience them for a long time and have substituted other tastes in their stead, we will eventually find that we no longer like those tastes. This is what has happened to me.

I found it very difficult at first when I stopped using sugar in my tea and coffee ... without resorting to artificial sweeteners. Nowadays I prefer sugarless tea and coffee and indeed I find drinking these with sugar very unpleasant. My taste buds have changed, have reverted to my pre-coffee and pre-tea drinking days.

Sweets (candies) and chocolates

Boiled sweets and candies, pastilles, jellied sweets, toffees, fudge, butterscotch, coconut bars, and a host of other sweets or candies including chocolates are usually loaded with fat and sugar which puts them all high up on the no-no list.

The only exception is black (or dark) chocolate, as studies have proved that this can be beneficial for cardiovascular health. In one study, regularly eating small amounts of dark chocolate was associated with a reduced risk of heart attacks.

However, as chocolate does contain plenty of fat it cannot help a diabetic unblock the receptors in muscle cells ... which is why I never eat more than one small square of dark chocolate a day.

Drinks

Sweetened drinks abound in our culture ... squashes, lemonades, sodas, sweetened fruit juices, various milk-based drinks and so on. These are all stamped on the no-no list.

What you can drink instead is plain water, mineral water, sugar- and milk-free tea or coffee, and a vast array of fruit and vegetable juices ... you'll soon acquire a taste for the latter.

Section Four: Outroduction

Diabetes is now epidemic, according to the Center for Disease Control, the National Institutes of Health, the American Diabetes Association and other national healthcare leaders ... Tim Holden

The purpose of this section is to summarise what needs to be done in order to beat diabetes.

Caveat: all the information in this book was obtained solely by research on the internet. It may not, therefore, be wholly accurate or I may have over-simplified some of the concepts. Nevertheless, the knowledge I gained through my research did help me to refine my diet so that I can go on beating my diabetes on a continuing basis.

31 - Cooking Tips

To succeed in beating your diabetes, you must only eat food that is low in fat, salt and sugar and has a high GI value.

Where fruit and vegetables are concerned finding foods that are low in fat is relatively easy ... only a few plants are high in fat and these have been mentioned in chapters 24, 25 and 30 so you can avoid them. In addition, if you are following the diet I am using to beat my diabetes, you have eliminated two main sources of fat from your diet ... eggs and dairy products.

You have also stopped eating processed meats. However you are still eating fresh meat and fish. To minimise your intake of fat you need to choose only lean meat and poultry and remove any fat you can see before cooking ... ie remove of the skin on chicken breasts, the rind on bacon, and the crackling on pork, etc, making sure you remove all visible traces of fat. And if any fat is visible when the meat is on your plate, you need to cut it out before you eat it.

Cooking is also very important ... you need to preserve the nutritional integrity of the food you are going to eat during cooking. This means ensuring that fat, salt and sugar are not added during the process and that vitamins are not destroyed by heat.

Here are a few broad tips which I have found useful.

Minimising oil
To beat your diabetes you need to minimise the oil you use in preparing your food. Here's how:

[1] Avoid the deep-fat fryer ... it is totally unnecessary and just adds fat to your food. Forget about chips, French fries, deep-fried chicken wings, battered fish and so on ... getting them off the menu won't cause any loss health wise.

[2] Use the grill rather than the frying pan ... but avoid brushing with oil before grilling, as it's not really necessary. Grilling is also beneficial because some of the fat in the food will drop off.

[3] Use a non-stick pan ... if you really must fry or sauté food, as q non-stick pan requires less oil than a standard frying pan.

[4] Use a cooking-spray ... to coat the ingredients in a thin film of oil before frying rather than pouring oil into the pan.

[5] Try using water instead of oil ... for frying or sautéing. It works sometimes, though not very well for me. However, I discovered that 'water-frying' works fine for vegetables.

[6] Steam-fry onions, garlic or vegetables ... in water or another liquid, instead of sautéing them in oil.

[7] Steam or boil vegetables ... rather than stir-frying them.

Avoiding salt

Being a diabetic you probably also, like me, have issues with your blood pressure. Thus you need to choose foods that contain little or no salt. As well as reading food labels closely, you should ensure that salt is not added during cooking.

Here's how ... use herbs, spices, and salt-free seasoning blends to add flavour, and ... cook rice, pasta, and hot cereals without adding any salt.

No added sugar

Since refined sugar was invented about 200 years ago the world as a whole, and Western culture in particular, has developed an incredibly sweet tooth. Sugar may be addictive (see chapter 12) but adding sugar during cooking is not necessary unless you are dealing with a fruit that is extremely tart (in which case I would suggest you eat something else).

You need to de-acquire your taste for sugar.

Cooking without sugar is easy. Where a recipe calls for sugar, just leave it out ... you can do this safely with most recipes. If the result is awful, don't cook that recipe again. There are thousands of other recipes you can follow.

For example, most recipes for pies and tarts call for sugar to be added to the fruit. I don't. You can make a very simple pie or tart using ordinary puff pastry and fresh or frozen fruit. Without sugar, the subtle flavours of the fruit come out and the taste is improved many times over.

Preserving vitamins

All of the water-soluble vitamins are easily lost during cooking ... they get washed out into the water in which the food is being boiled.

The best way to preserve vitamins when cooking is to use as little water as possible and cook the food (usually vegetables) for as short a time as possible. Also, save the cooking water (which is bound to contain some washed out vitamins) to use in other food such as a soup or low-fat gravy.

If you need to add iron to your diet, cook your food in a cast-iron pan (skillet) or pot ... a tiny bit of the iron will come off and mix with the food.

Glycemic index

To beat your diabetes it is important that you eat food that is digested slowly, ie that has low glycemic index values and so releases glucose into your bloodstream slowly. The problem is that cooking can raise the GI values of particular foods.

Pasta, for example, has a low glycemic index. This is because uncooked pasta has no air-pockets ... which means your digestive juices cannot get at the molecules of semolina quickly to break them down. But you must stop the cooking while the pasta is still al-dente (chewy). If you overcook it, it will expand, develop air-pockets and be digested rapidly. The longer you cook pasta, the more its GI value rises.

Other foodstuffs act similarly ... overcooking raises GI and speeds up the rate at which glucose is released into your bloodstream.

The take-away is ... do NOT overcook ... any food ... ever.

Cooking beans

As you will be eating a plant-focused diet and because beans are known to deliver more protein than other plants, you need to make them a core part of your food-stocks.

While you will probably rely on tinned or commercially prepared beans initially, it is well to know how to cook beans from scratch.

Fresh beans in their pods (haricots verts etc) are cooked just like any other vegetable. Shelled beans, however, are usually bought dried. Dried beans and legumes, with the exceptions of black-eyed peas and lentils, need to be rehydrated by soaking them in water at room-temperature water before they can be cooked.

There are several ways you can soak beans. But before soaking, you need to 'clean them up' by sorting through the beans and discarding any discoloured or shrivelled ones or any foreign matter. It's best to soak beans overnight.

Put half a kilogram of dried beans in a large pot, add 2.5 litres (10 cups) of cold water, cover and refrigerate for eight hours. A quicker way is to bring the water to the boil, add the beans, bring the water back to boiling, remove from the heat, cover tightly and let it sit at room temperature for about three hours. If you are in a rush, you can save two hours if you re-boil the beans for two or three minutes before setting them aside.

If beans give you flatulence, you can get rid of most of the indigestible sugars that cause the gas by using the last method mentioned in the previous paragraph ... but instead of setting them aside for only an hour after boiling for two or three minutes, let them stand overnight. The next day you'll find that 75 percent of the sugars that cause gas will have dissolved into the water and you can get rid of them by discarding this water and using fresh water to cook the beans.

After soaking, rinse the beans and put them in a large pot. Cover them with three times their volume of water. Add herbs or spices as you like, and bring to the boil. Then reduce the heat and simmer them gently, uncovered, stirring occasionally, until they are tender. Add more water if the beans become uncovered.

The cooking time depends on the type of bean, but they usually take at least 45 minutes. Beans are done when they can be easily mashed between two fingers or with a fork.

If you want to add salt (which you shouldn't) or acidic ingredients, such as vinegar or tomato juice, wait until near the end of the cooking time, when the beans are just tender. If you add them too early, they will probably make the beans tough and slow down the cooking.

Brown rice

When I first switched to eating brown (whole) rice instead of white rice, I could never get it right. I would cook it the same way as I used to cook white rice, ie boiling it gently in twice its volume of water.

Once most of the water had gone, I would have nice fluffy white rice. But with this method, brown rice always ended up gritty and too hard to chew.

Then I discovered the secret of brown rice ... cook it the same way as you would cook pasta ... using plenty of water and then draining the excess water once the rice is cooked.

32 - Checklist -1: Monitoring

The diet I have outlined in this book worked for me. Thus it should also work for you ... enable you to beat your diabetes and avoid the horrendous consequences of this pernicious disease.

However, in order to be sure your diet is working, you need to monitor your health as indicated in the first few chapters of this book. If you don't do so, you'll be 'flying blind' ... you won't know whether your diet is being effective or not.

Another good reason to monitor 'your numbers' is the satisfaction of watching your numbers fall.

Here's a summary of what you have to keep your eye on. The numbers in brackets in the sub-titles refer to the chapters in which these matters are discussed.

Insulin sensitivity (chapter 3)
Your body's sensitivity to insulin, ie how well insulin can open the receptors in your muscle cells and allow glucose to enter those cells, is what defines you as a diabetic. It is measured using two indicators.

Blood glucose levels ... ideally you should monitor your blood glucose four times a day ... when you awake in the morning and two hours after each meal. Aim for levels of 5–7 mmol/l (90–126 mg/dl).

Consistent readings above this range would be a cause for concern ... you should review your diet. If being more stringent in the elimination of fat from your diet does not result in blood glucose levels that fall within the range then you should consult your doctor or diabetes clinic.

HbA1c ... you should also have the main indicator as to how well you are managing your diabetes checked three times a year. You should aim for HbA1c levels that are less than 48 mmol/mol (6.5%).

Blood pressure (chapter 5)
If you have diabetes but are not yet hypertensive, you should have your blood pressure checked regularly, say four times a year.

If you both diabetic and hypertensive, you should monitor and record your blood pressure at home. Aim for pressures below 115/75mmHg ... with 112/64mmHg as an ultimate target. You should also take your prescribed medications, exercise regularly, not smoke, and reduce the salt in your diet.

Cholesterol & Triglycerides (chapter 6)

As you are diabetic, there is an 85% chance that you also have issues with your cholesterol.

As well as taking any prescribed medicines, you should have your cholesterol and triglycerides levels checked regularly, at least twice a year.

Your target levels should be:

LDL cholesterol ... no more than 1.8mmol/l (70mg/dl) ... but try for 1.0mmol/l (40mg/dl)
HDL cholesterol (for **men**) ... above 1.2mmol/l (45mg/dl)
HDL cholesterol (for **women**)... above 1.4mmol/l (55mg/dl)
Cholesterol ratio ... 1:3 (ratio of HDL to total cholesterol)
Triglycerides ... less than 1.69mmol/l (150mg/dl)

Weight (chapter 9)

To help maintain your body's sensitivity to insulin, you need to control your weight, ie, you need to measure and record your weight once a week. Each time you weigh yourself, you should also calculate you BMI (divide your body weight in kilograms by the square of your height in metres).

If you are overweight or obese, ie if your BMI is over 25 (or 23 if you are East Asian), use your BMI Prime figure (your actual BMI divided by 25 or 23) to calculate how much you are overweight ... this will indicate how much weight you need to lose.

Then employ a combination of reduced food intake and increased exercising to return your BMI to the normal range.

Feet (chapter 9)

Check your feet daily for signs of injury or infection and have any problems attended to immediately. You should also have your feet examined by a doctor once a year and tested for sensitivity.

To protect your feet (always a problem for diabetics), do not walk barefoot, even around the house. You should also ensure that your shoes are loose-fitting and do not pinch or squeeze your feet.

Skin (chapter 2)
Once a day you should examine your skin, especially your legs, for signs of injury or infection.

Eyes (chapter 2)
Diabetes can cause several serious problems to your eyes, so you should have your eyes dilated and examined by an ophthalmologist once a year.

Exercise (chapter 8)
In my experience, diet is more important than exercise in beating diabetes. Nevertheless, exercising regularly is necessary for controlling your blood pressure, cholesterol and triglycerides, with which you most likely have issues as you are diabetic. Exercising is a cinch:

Start the day with mild stretching or flexibility exercises, ie a morning limber-up as described in chapter 8. You should also get in some aerobic exercising ... a daily 30-minute walk is fine, which you can break up into three shorter walks if you wish. And a few push-ups or sit-ups once a day will deliver all the anaerobic exercising you may need.

However, if you have diabetic neuropathy and wish to try to reverse you symptoms, you'll need a much more vigorous exercise regime.

Smoking (chapter 7)
Smoking is for schmucks (like me). Don't smoke.

If you do, give it up ... do whatever it takes to kill your habit ... permanently

Note: you can download a handy checklist on monitoring your health from www.beating-diabetes.com. Just go to DOWNLOADS in the right sidebar and click on *Signup and download Checklists & References*.

33 - Checklist -2: Diet

Eat natural ... low sugar ... low fat ... low salt ... high fibre ... low GI ... mostly plants ... and drink lots of water

Natural ... choose fresh or frozen food rather than processed foodstuffs.

Sugar ... reduce consumption as far as possible ... beware of added sugar in sweetened foodstuffs ... all beverages should be sugar-free

Fat ... restrict intake to 2–3% by weight of solid food and, for liquid foods, to 10% of calories from fat

Salt ... limit your salt intake to 1.15–2.3g (0.2 - 0.4 teaspoon) of salt (0.46–0.92g (0.05 - 0.1 teaspoon) of sodium) a day

Fibre ... include 40g a day in your diet and drink plenty of water

Glycemic index ... eat foods that have low GI values

Mostly plants ... focus your choices of foodstuffs on legumes, vegetables and fruits

Water ... drink at least 4 litres (135oz) a day of water including all other beverages (tea, coffee, juices, etc) ... keep a large jug of water on your desk to make this easier

If the above seems daunting ... it isn't.

No measuring of quantities is involved ... in fact, if you learn to read labels (chapter 34) and just eat the 'Allowed' foodstuffs in the listings below, you will be automatically following these guidelines.

Supplements
I take each day:
- Multivitamin tablet
- Vitamin B12 (4mcg) tablet

- Calcium (400mg) tablet with vitamin D (2.5mcg)
- Cod Liver oil capsule that includes vitamins D and E
- Cinnamon (one large teaspoon on cereal)

The supplements you choose to take should match your own particular needs. However, a multivitamin tablet is necessary as you have eliminated a whole food group, dairy products, as well as eggs, from your diet.

Grains (chapters 20 and 21)

Grains consist of dinner grains, breakfast cereals, breads, pastries and cakes.

The basic rule is ... choose wholemeal rather than refined grains

Dinner grains (chapter 30)

Eat regularly:

Rice (brown)
Barley (hulled)
Rye berries
Semolina (savoury, not sweet)
Bulgur wheat
Couscous
Noodles (made from whole-grains only)
Pasta (unleavened, wholemeal, cooked al-dente)
Millet (only a little or occasionally - nutrients difficult to digest)

Note: eat pasta only if it is cooked al-dente (otherwise its GI value is high)

Avoid:

Rice (white)
Barley (pearl or pearled)
Noodles (made from refined grains)
Malts (malted grains)
Pasta (well cooked)
Pasta (made with eggs)

Breakfast cereals (chapter 30)

Eat regularly:

Whole-meal porridge (oatmeal) made from rolled oats
Oat Bran (add to porridge)
Cold cereals (whole-grain, no added sugar)
Muesli (home-made without nuts)

Avoid:
Instant / quick porridge or oatmeal (high GI)
Children's cereals (high sugar)
Coco Pops (high sugar)
Clusters (high sugar)
Commercial muesli (high sugar, nuts)

Bread (chapter 21)
Eat regularly
Wholemeal breads
Rye breads (eg pumpernickel)
Crisp breads made from rye
Unleavened flatbreads (but check for salt)
Roti (unleavened whole-wheat Indian bread)
Chapatti (unleavened whole-wheat Indian bread)
Malt loaf (but only if it is sugar-free)

Eat very little
Wheat-germ bread (white bread with added wheat-germ)
Granary bread (contains some white flour)
Whole-grain bread (white bread with added whole grains)

Avoid
White bread
Brown bread (coloured white bread)
Quick breads (unless made from wholemeal flour)
Irish soda bread (unless made from wholemeal flour)
Breads with high salt content
Breads made with shortening, unless fat is less than 3% by weight
Fried breads
Puri (Indian fried bread)
Malted breads (sugar)

Pastries (chapter 30)

Due to their high fat and sugar content, pastries are out of bounds with the occasional exception of simple pastries combined with plain fruit.

Eat maximum once a week:
Fruit-filled pies made with simple pastry with no added sugar

Avoid:
Danish pastries (fat, sugar)
Croissant (fat, sugar)
Brioche (fat, egg)
Mille-feuille (sugar, pastry cream)
Profiteroles (sugar, pastry cream)
Cream puffs (sugar, pastry cream)
Choux a la creme (sugar, pastry cream)
Eclairs (sugar, pastry cream)

Cakes (chapters 21 and 30)
Avoid:
All cakes (fat, sugar)
Semolina products (unless they are sugar-free)

Legumes (chapter 22)
Eat plenty;
Beans, especially:
- Black beans
- Pinto beans
- Navy beans (as in baked beans)
Peas
Chickpeas (choose Desi (lower GI) rather than Kabuli)
Lentils (green lentils for more fibre)
Textured vegetable protein (textured soy protein)

Eat reasonable quantities:
Tofu in savoury dishes
Tempeh (soy cake)
Sweet or dessert tofu (check for added sugar)
Miso soup (in moderation)

Avoid:
Peanuts (fat)

Soya beans (fat)
Miso (salt)

Soya and soy products
Use regularly:
Soy milk - excellent substitute for animal milk

Eat with caution:
Soy yoghurt - check labels for added sweeteners

Avoid:
Soya beans (fat)
Soy cheese (fat)
Soy sauce (salt, carcinogens)

Vegetables (chapter 24)
Frozen or fresh are best
Tinned vegetables - check labels for added sugar

Eat regularly
Tomatoes (one a day)
Crucifers (cabbage family)
- Cabbage
- Brussels sprouts
- Broccoli
- Cauliflower
- Turnips
- Kale
- Bak choy
Artichokes (improves glucose levels)
Celery (lowers blood pressure and cholesterol levels)
Spinach (good for arteries)
Lettuce (maintain weight)
Bell peppers (prefer red to green)
Onions and garlic (as much as possible - helps metabolic syndrome)
Mushrooms (twice a week)

Eat regularly in moderation

Roots, bulbs and tubers (energy-dense)
Carrots (one a day at least)
Radishes
Sweet potatoes (low-GI)
Yams (low-GI)

Eat with caution
Potatoes (high GI)
Roast potatoes (fat, high GI)

Avoid (high fat content)
Olives (fat 15-30%)
Avocado (fat 15%)
Chips (French fries)
Crisps (chips)

Fruit (chapter 25)
Consume a minimum of three pieces of fruit (including juice and dried fruit) a day
Dried fruit - only eat about 1/3 of amount of fresh fruit you'd eat - but first check whether sugar was infused before drying.

Eat regularly
Apple (one a day - eat skin but not pips)
Pear (substitute for daily apple)
Blackberries (less sugar than other fruit)
Raspberries (lots of fibre)
Bananas - one-a-day maximum (sugar)
Apricots - dried are preferable (lower GI and concentrated nutrients)

Eat in moderation
Blackcurrants
Redcurrants
Gooseberries
Guava

Eat only a little
Banana (one a day max - sugar)

Peaches and nectarines (sugar, relatively high GI)
Cranberries (sugar)
Strawberries (sugar)
Pomegranates (sugar)
Melon (sugar)
Kiwifruit (sugar)
Papaya (sugar)
Grapes (sugar 15%)
Watermelon (high GI)
Pineapple (high GI)
Cherries (high sugar, low GI)
Blueberries (high sugar, high fibre)
Dried fruit (sun/hot-air dried) - limit consumption to 1/3 of fresh fruit equivalent

Avoid

Dates (fresh - sugar 60%)
Figs (fresh - sugar 48%)
Coconut (fat 33.5%)
Açaí (fat 32.5%)
Plums and prunes (except as laxative)
Crystallised fruits (candied or glacé fruit, such as dates, cherries, pineapple, ginger, chestnuts (marron glacé), orange peel and lemon peel)
Dried fruit (sugar-infused before drying)
Tinned (canned) fruit (with added sugar)
Grapefruit (adversely interferes with metabolism of vital drugs)
Other citrus fruits - treat with extreme caution until effect on metabolism of vital drugs assessed

Fruit juices (chapter 25)
Allowed

1/2 glass of any fruit juice a day (provided unsweetened)
Apple juice (check for added sugar)

Avoid

Fruit juices with added sugar
Blackcurrant juice (always has sugar added)
Redcurrant juice (always has sugar added)

Grapefruit juice (interferes with metabolism of vital drugs)
Other citrus juices (until effect on metabolism of vital drugs assessed)

Fruit products (chapter 30)
Eat very occasionally
Jam (made without sugar) but use thin smear (only) on toast

Avoid
Jams (commercial - fat, sugar)
Desserts (commercial - fat, sugar)
Pies and crumbles (commercial - fat, sugar)
Gooseberry products (always have sugar added)

Nuts (chapter 30)
Avoid
All nuts (fat 40-70%)

Occasional treat
Almonds (good for cholesterol)
Walnuts (good for cholesterol)

Eggs (chapter 28)
Avoid
Eliminate eggs 100% from your diet

Dairy (chapter 29)
Avoid
Eliminate ALL dairy products 100% from your diet, including:
- Milk (fat, cholesterol, sugar, animal protein)
- Yoghurt (fat, cholesterol, sugar)
- Cheese (fat, cholesterol, sugar)
- Sour cream (fat, cholesterol, sugar)
- Ice cream (fat, cholesterol, sugar)
- Butter (fat, cholesterol, salt)
Casein (milk protein) - you need to check non-dairy products for the presence of casein.

Dairy substitutes

Soy milk (instead of cows or goats milk)
Oat milk (instead of cows or goats milk)
Rice milk (instead of cows or goats milk)
Almond milk (instead of cows or goats milk)
Vegan ice cream (check for added sugar)
Vegetarian products (check for sugar, fat, casein, egg whites)

Processed meats (chapter 30)
Avoid
All processed meats (salt, nitrates, sugar etc)
Bacon (fat)
Sausages (fat)
Black and white puddings (fat)

Occasional treat
Boiled ham - provided salt used in curing extracted by soaking before cooking

Allowed
Dried lean meat (eg, biltong, beef jerky) but only if not salted

Unprocessed animal products
Allowed
Red meat - small ultra-lean amounts
Chicken (remove skin) - small ultra-lean amounts
Turkey (remove skin) - small ultra-lean amounts
Fish (remove skin) - small amounts

Snacks
Allowed
Fruit
Raw vegetables
Smoothies made of fresh fruit and vegetables, soy milk (or similar) provided no added sugar

Avoid
Confectionary - all

Fats and oils (chapter 30)

Only use vegetable oils but restrict to 2–3% of daily calorific intake (= max fat needed by body)

Minimal use
    Corn oil
    Sunflower oil
    Soy oil
    Safflower oil
    Rapeseed oil
    Olive oil (13% saturated fat)

Avoid
    Suet
    Dripping

Sauces, dressings and condiments (chapter 30)

For all packaged sauces, dressings and condiments ... ensure that less than 10% calories come from fat or they only have 2 or 3g fat per serving

Allowed
    Tabasco sauce (but check labels for fat, sugar and salt)
    Worcestershire sauce (but check labels for fat, sugar and salt)
    Lemon juice
    Balsamic vinegar
    Fat-free dressings for salads
    Vinaigrettes (home-made without oil)
    Pickles (but check labels for fat, sugar and salt)
    Chutneys (but check labels for fat, sugar and salt)
    Spices and herbs

Treat with caution
    Vinaigrettes (commercial, provided very little fat)

Avoid
    Redcurrant sauce (sugar)
    Redcurrant jelly (sugar)
    Soy sauce (salt, carcinogens)
    Salad dressing (fat)

Mayonnaise (fat)
Dressings with oil

Jams, preserves and spreads (chapter 30)

Most jams and preserves contain excessive sugar, while most spreads are fat-heavy.

Allowed
    Jams (made without sugar) - use extremely sparingly
    Marmalades (made without sugar) - use extremely sparingly
    Marmite - check labels
    Bovril - check labels

Avoid
    Butter (fat)
    Margarine (fat 80%)
    Honey (sugar 99%)
    Jams (sugar)
    Marmalades (sugar)

Artificial sweeteners (chapter 30)

Avoid
    Artificial sweeteners (to retrain taste-buds)

Sweets (candies) and chocolates (chapter 30)

Basically, all types of sweets (candies) and chocolates are off, with one exception

Allowed
    Dark chocolate (maximum one square a day - fat)

Avoid
    Boiled sweets / candies (sugar)
    Pastilles (sugar)
    Jellied sweets (sugar)
    Toffees (fat, sugar)
    Fudge (fat, sugar)
    Butterscotch (fat, sugar)
    Coconut bars (fat, sugar)

Chocolates (fat, sugar)

Drinks
Drink copiously
> Water (plain) - minimum 2 to 4 litres a day
> Water (mineral) - drink all you want

Drink regularly
> Tea (sugar-free)
> Coffee (sugar-free)
> Fruit juices (no added sugar) - 1/2 glass a day
> Vegetable juices (no added sugar) - 1 glass a day

Avoid
> Squashes (sugar)
> Lemonades (sugar)
> Sodas (sugar)
> Sweetened fruit juices (sugar)
> Milk-based drinks (dairy, sugar)

Note: you can download a handy checklist on your diabetes-beating diet from www.beating-diabetes.com. Just go to DOWNLOADS in the right sidebar and click on *Signup and download Checklists & References.*

34 - Shopping

My purpose in writing this book was to show you how I am managing (so far at least) to beat my type 2 diabetes and give you the basic knowledge you need in order to beat your diabetes.

Hopefully you now know how to monitor your condition, what to do to prevent this incurable disease from developing, the type of diet you should follow and, most importantly, an outline of the contents (nutritious or otherwise) present in various common foodstuffs.

Now that you know what foods you should be eating, you need to go out and buy them. But first you have to do a bit of exploring ... find out where you can get the foods that will exactly fit your diet.

You should start, as I did, by exploring your local supermarket and health-food stores to see what they offer. Get to know the bread, fruit and vegetable sections. Check out the butchery for ultra-lean fresh meat. You may be able to find Chinese, Thai or Japanese food in your local supermarket. If so, you will surely discover plenty of healthful plant-based foods. If not, visit the nearest ethnic stores.

Most major supermarkets have health-food and dietetic sections and you should be able to find plenty of products you can use. However, be cautious when it comes to food for dieters ... these may be low in fat but high in sugar. Conversely, food intended for diabetics can be equally bad ... low in sugar but often high in fats.

Exploring your local food stores and deciding what you can eat only requires a little time and one simple skill ... the ability to read food labels.

Indeed, as most of the foods we buy (the exceptions being fresh fruit, vegetables and meats) consist of processed foods, becoming adept at reading food labels is vital for beating your diabetes.

How else could you make informed purchases?

Food labels

Most countries in the developed world have stringent requirements as to what goes into foodstuffs and what must be shown on the packaging. Besides the name of the food and its type, and the name and address of the manufacturer, the label usually includes:
- net quantity;

- list of the ingredients; and
- nutritional information.

The net quantity ... is the amount of food (by weight or volume) contained within the package, ie excluding the container but including any water or liquid. For foods where the liquid is discarded by the consumer (such as olives) the drained weight is usually also shown.

In Europe, the net quantity is shown as the weight (usually grams) or volume (litres or millilitres). In the USA, the net quantity is also shown as ounces, pounds or fluid ounces.

In both hemispheres, the weight is shown for solid and mixed solid-liquid foods, while the volume is used for liquid foods.

The ingredients listing ... shows the common names for the ingredients. In the USA these are listed in descending order by weight or volume, ie the heaviest or largest is shown first.

The list also includes items such as flavourings, colourings, preservatives, and humectants (which help products retain water). But where an ingredient comprises less than 2% of the total weight or volume it may be shown as 'contains less than 2% of ...

As an example, here's a list of typical ingredients for wholemeal tortillas ... wholemeal wheat flour, water, vegetable oil, humectant (glycerine), raising agents (diphosphates, sodium bicarbonate), dextrose, salt, acidity regulators (malic acid, citric acid), preservative (calcium propionate), emulsifier (mono- and diglycerides of fatty acids).

Ingredients that have a specific function, such as preservatives, must also have their function shown. In Europe the nature of the ingredient is listed first with the actual ingredient following immediately in brackets, eg humectant (glycerine). In the USA, this is reversed and the actual ingredient is shown with the functional nature in brackets, viz, glycerine (humectant).

Ingredients that are made up of other ingredients (such as sauces) are still listed in their place in the descending order but are immediately followed by a list (inside brackets) of each ingredient they, in turn, contain.

For example, if a product contains tomato sauce, it will be listed as (say) ... potatoes, tomato sauce (tomatoes, vinegar, sugar, onions, garlic and celery), garlic, etc...

Nutritional information ... consists of all the macro-nutrients and many of the micro-nutrients a food provides and is usually displayed in a box format.

The information includes the quantity of each nutrient per 100g or per 100ml, and per serving. The size of serving is also shown, eg 10g, 30cl.

The information in the box usually begins with the number of calories, followed by the calories from fat. Then the amount of protein, fat, saturated fat, trans-fat, cholesterol, carbohydrates, sugar, fibre, and sodium are usually listed with their quantities.

Micro-nutrients such as vitamin A, vitamin C, calcium, and iron may be shown separately at the bottom of the box.

Insignificant amounts of nutrients, ie those that weight less than 1 gram or for which the quantity expressed as a decimal would round to zero, are usually left out of the nutritional information even though they appear in the list of ingredients. Examples include various spices.

Healthful claims

The packages of many food products often proclaim that the products concerned have special attributes that make for healthful eating. Examples include 'low salt', 'sugar free' and so on.

The regulations in the European Union do not contain legal definitions of terms such as 'low fat' or 'high fibre', though terms such as 'reduced calories' may not be used unless the product can be shown to be significantly lower in calories than its original version.

Americans consumers are much more fortunate. In the USA food-labelling regulations place clearly defined limits on the meanings of specific terms such as 'free', 'low', 'lean', 'extra lean', 'high', 'good source', 'reduced', 'less', 'light', 'more' and 'healthy'.

Free ... refers to products that contain trivial (but not necessarily zero) amounts of a nutrient. For example, sugar-free and fat-free both mean less than 0.5g per serving, while calorie-free means less than 5 calories per serving. The same rule applies to terms such as 'without', 'no', and 'zero'.

Low ... refers to foods that can be eaten often without breaking the dietary guidelines for calories, fat, saturated fat, cholesterol, and sodium. Other terms and phrases such as 'little', 'few', 'low source of ...', and 'contains a small amount of ...' fall under the same rules as 'low'.

These rules are:

Low-calorie ... 40 calories or less per serving

Low-fat ... max 3g per serving

Low-saturated fat ... max 1g per serving

Low-cholesterol ... max 20mg of cholesterol and max 2g of saturated fat per serving

Low-sodium ... max 140mg per serving

Very-low-sodium ... max 35mg per serving

And, of course, the size of the serving must be shown on the package.

Lean and extra lean ... refer to the fat in red meat, game, poultry, and seafood. They are defined as:

Lean ... max 10g of fat, max 4.5g of saturated fat, and less than 95mg cholesterol in a single serving or 100g (whichever is lower)

Extra lean ... less than 5g of fat, less than 2g of saturated fat, and less than 95mg cholesterol in a single serving or 100g (whichever is lower).

Less ... refers to a food that contains 25% fewer calories or 25% less of a particular nutrient than the original or reference food.

Reduced ... refers to a food that contains more than 25% fewer calories or more than 25% less of a particular nutrient than the reference food.

Light ... refers to a product that contains one-third fewer calories or half the fat of the reference food.

Light in sodium ... means that the sodium content has been reduced by at least 50%.

Dietary guidelines

Dietary guidelines consist of recommended amounts of macro- and micro-nutrients that should be consumed daily by a healthy person who is over four years of age.

In the USA and Canada these are known as dietary values or reference daily intakes (RDIs), while in Europe they are called guideline daily amounts (GDAs) when they relate to macro-nutrients and recommended daily allowances (RDAs) when they refer to vitamins and dietary minerals.

The guidelines are based on a diet of 2000 calories a day that is sufficient to meet the dietary requirements all healthy persons. Each serving of food you eat will deliver a portion of the amounts of the various macro-nutrients (proteins, fats, carbohydrates and sodium) as well as a portion of the various amounts of micro-nutrients (vitamins and minerals) you need on a daily basis.

The portion of each nutrient is shown as a percentage under nutritional information. For each nutrient, the percentage of the daily value delivered by a serving or 100 grams of the particular food is shown.

For example, according to the guidelines, you should eat 65g of total fat a day. If a serving of a particular food gives you 15g of fat, then next to the 15g you'll see 23%, ie if you eat one serving of that food you will have ingested 23% of your daily requirement for fat.

The utility of these guidelines and their relevance to health is disputed among nutritionists and between nations. For example, the recommended intakes for some nutrients (such as sodium) differ sharply between the USA and the UK.

Personally, I feel that catch-all single figure recommendations to cover all members of a population (except infants) do not make sense. Surely the dietary needs of an athletic healthy young man are quite different from the requirements of a sedentary widow in her late 80s? And just as surely, won't those of us who have long-term illnesses such as diabetes have very different dietary needs from the average healthy person?

About 6% of the populations of North America and Europe have diabetes ... would 65g of fat a day help them unblock the receptors in their muscle cells and beat the disease? I think not.

For these reasons, and also for the fact that it would be impossible to record all the nutrients you eat everyday, I ignore these guidelines.

I feel that if I follow a plant-focused diet that is low in sugar, fat and salt, is high in fibre and the consists mainly of natural unprocessed food with low GI values, along with plenty of water, I should be doing OK as regards macro-nutrients.

And I'm quite sure that popping a comprehensive multi-vitamin each day takes care of the micro-nutrients I need.

Reading food labels

To read food labels, you just check the list of ingredients and the nutrition facts.

Ingredients list ... I just make sure that there are (a) no animal-derived ingredients, (b) no partially hydrogenated vegetable oils (aka trans-fats), and (c) no or only a little added sugar.

In the diet I am following to beat my diabetes, I do eat some fresh ultra-lean meat and fish. All the same I ensure, out of deference to my kidneys and because I do not eat eggs or dairy products at all, that the processed foods I eat do not contain any animal products.

Common, animal-derived ingredients include ... milk solids ... whey ... casein (and casein derivatives, eg sodium caseinate) ... egg products ... gelatine, and ... cheese. With these in mind, I peruse the ingredients list closely.

Nutrition facts ... once I am satisfied that the ingredients in the food product are acceptable, I check to see whether the product meets my nutritional needs.

Ideally, a serving will contain ... a maximum of 2 grams of fat ... a maximum of 10% energy from fat, and ... no cholesterol. If it does contain any cholesterol then it must contain animal-derived ingredients as plants do not contain any cholesterol.

It should also be low in sodium (salt) and have a low glycemic index value, though this will not be shown under nutrition facts. However, if the glycemic index value is low, this may be shown (usually prominently) on the package itself.

I also try to ensure that a particular food has low energy-density, ie less than one calorie per gram. You can easily work this out in your head by taking the total calories in 100g and dividing by 100 (ie moving the decimal point two places). For example, a 100g of a typical wholemeal tortilla will give you 273 calories; thus the energy-density is 2.73 calories per gram (which is too high).

It's quite difficult to find processed foods where the energy-density is less than one calorie per gram. However I don't think the energy density is anything to get hung up about and as long as the energy-density is reasonable you should be OK.

Once you have found what you need to support your diabetes-beating diet, you don't have to go looking again ... you only have to read the labels on new products that you have not yet considered.

Reading labels only applies to processed products that contain more than one ingredient or are canned. Single ingredient foods, such as cuts of fresh meat and fish, vegetables and fruit, are not labelled. As you are going on a plant-focused diet, you won't have too much label reading to do.

Note: you can download a handy checklist on reading food labels from www.beating-diabetes.com. Just go to DOWNLOADS in the right sidebar and click on *Signup and download Checklists & References.*

END

Afterword

I hope you enjoyed reading *Beating Diabetes* and found it beneficial. I'm sure you now realise that avoiding the horrendous consequences of type 2 diabetes is easy ... all you have to do is change your diet and make a few minor adjustments to your lifestyle. Nothing could be simpler; and you don't need a great deal of will-power either.

To help, you can download a booklet of handy checklists and other material from www.beating-diabetes.com. The contents include:

- Checklist for monitoring diabetes
- Checklist for a diabetes-beating diet
- Conversion chart
- Fibre check
- Table of GI values
- Dietary guidelines
- Reading food labels

Just go to www.beating-diabetes.com and look for DOWNLOADS in the right side-bar. Click on *Signup and download Checklists & References* which will take you to a sign-up form. After signing up you will receive an email with a link to *Checklists & References* which you can open and then save to your hard disk.

If you have any comments, queries or suggestions, or discover any mistakes that need correcting, please email me on: paul@beating-diabetes.com

Paul Kennedy writes a weekly blog on topics of interest for type 2 diabetics. To put yourself on the mailing list for these articles, just to go to www.beating-diabetes.com and click on SIGN-UP.

Privacy policy: please note that we will never share your email address with anyone at all. You can read our full privacy policy on our website: www.beating-diabetes.com.

Paul D Kennedy is an international business consultant, researcher, writer and publisher. He is a graduate of Trinity College, Dublin, and a Fellow of the Chartered Association of Certified Accountants. *Beating Diabetes* is based on his own personal experience in avoiding the horrendous consequence of type 2 diabetes. You can contact Paul at:

paul@beating-diabetes.com

Websites
www.beating-diabetes.com
www.thornislandpublishing.com
www.consulting-services.eu
www.writingservices.eu
www.kuwaitbusinessguide.com
www.kuwait1990.com
www.arabic-tales.com

26256947R00156

Made in the USA
Charleston, SC
31 January 2014